NEW FACTS ABOUT

FIBER

Health Builder
Disease Fighter
Vital Nutrient

How Fiber Supplements
Enhance Your Health

by Betty Kamen, Ph.D..

Nutrition Encounter, Inc., Novato, California

All of the facts in this book have been very carefully re-searched, and have been drawn from the scientific literature. In no way, however, are any of the suggestions meant to take the place of advice given by physicians. Please consult a medical or health professional should the need for one be indicated.

First printing: 1991
Second printing: 1991
Third printing: 1992
Fourth printing: 1992
Fifth printing: 1994

Printed in the United States of America
ISBN 0-944501-05-2

Dedicated to:

Denis Burkitt, M.D.

observant researcher
who, more than a decade ago, introduced
fiber concepts
in this country
to my listening audience
and to me
in the
studios of WMCA, New York

CONTENTS

Recipes

Tables

Medical Conditions Discussed in Chapter 3

OTHER BOOKS BY BETTY KAMEN, Ph.D..

Total Nutrition During Pregnancy:
How To Be Sure You and Your Baby
Are Eating the Right Stuff

Total Nutrition for Breast-Feeding Mothers

Kids Are What They Eat:
What Every Parent Needs to Know About Nutrition

In Pursuit of Youth: Everyday Nutrition

Osteoporosis:
What It Is, How to Prevent It, How to Stop It

Nutrition In Nursing: The New Approach
A Handbook of Nursing Science

Sesame: The Superfood Seed
How It Can Add Vitality To Your Life

Siberian Ginseng:
Up-To-Date Research on the Fabled Tonic Herb

Germanium: A New Approach to Immunity

Startling New Facts About Osteoporosis:
Why Calcium Alone Does Not Prevent Bone Disease

The Chromium Diet, Supplement & Exercise Strategy

Everything You Always Wanted to Know About Potassium
But Were Too Tired to Ask

Betty Kamen is an award-winning photojournalist, with graduate degrees in psychology and nutrition education. She is an internationally-known lecturer, radio/TV host, and the author of many major books, hundreds of articles, and several tapes on various aspects of health and nutrition. For many years, she hosted *Nutrition 57* on WMCA in New York, followed by *Nutrition Watch* on KNBR in San Francisco.

ACKNOWLEDGMENTS

Larry Jordan, for planting seeds of knowledge

Si Kamen, for support and commitment

Jarrow (Rogavin), Peter Finkel, Theresa James,
Bernice Goldmark, and Brad Opstad
for refining judgment,
clarifying language,
and challenging concepts

Perle Kinney, for being there

FOREWORD

Most people need to be made aware that fiber is not just another food fad and that we could improve our fiber intake through a better knowledge of fiber sources. The discrepancies between dietary guidelines and our actual diets suggest a great urgency for this kind of education. Clarifications of fiber concepts, as outlined in Betty Kamen's book, provide a powerful stimulus for diet change.

The dietary fiber consumption of the average person in our country is only one-fifth of what it was a hundred years ago, and the consequences have been overwhelmingly disastrous. Health or illness depends on a balance between factors that *cause* and those that *protect against* the development of disease. The lack or availability of fiber in our diets is a major determinant of that balance.

Fiber is a complex substance. Equally complex is our search for understanding exactly how and why fiber helps to alleviate, and even prevent, so many nutritionally-linked diseases. The extensive documentation in this book places us on a sounder footing toward comprehending the fiber/disease paradigm.

Since different fibers initiate different responses, it is advisable to obtain adequate fiber from a wide variety of sources rather than excessive amounts from a single source, as Dr. Kamen reports. This also minimizes the possibility of food sensitivity, which often occurs with an overconsumption of a single food substance.

Most physicians are engaged in *intervention*—advice and treatment for the management of degenerative disease, and in *therapy*—advice intended to reduce risk of recurrence after treatment for disease. But *prevention*, advice for the general population, is often neglected. *New Facts About Fiber* fills the missing gap. The recommendations on dietary intake are transmitted in a form that allows for ready application. Although we are much more knowledgeable about nutrition than ever before, diet behavior is not consistent with nutrition knowledge. Dr. Kamen addresses this issue with realistic insights and solutions.

Stephen E. Langer, M.D.
Berkeley, California

AUTHOR'S NOTES

AWAKENINGS

When Denis Burkitt, a British surgeon studying the diets of rural Africans, compared the size of hospitals with the size of the end product of our *digesta* more than ten years ago, he initiated a fiber renaissance. His discovery?

Large stools, small hospitals; small stools, large hospitals.

And, like Topsy, the fiber revival just "growed." So it is that *high fiber* has replaced *bland* on the physician's prescription pad, and so it is that we have been bombarded with information. Endless books on the virtues of consuming more healthful food has even reached New York Times best-seller status. But America's eating habits have not been altered in any meaningful way! If it isn't lack of information, what's wrong?

Several hundred people in four grocery stores were questioned during a recent survey. "Let's find out," the researchers said, "what people really know about fiber." It turns out that consumers are somewhat familiar with the role fiber may play in the prevention or treatment of certain diseases or conditions. They get an F, however, when it comes to fiber sources and recommended intake. Consumers do not appear to understand how to translate health messages into usable information. Fiber knowledge gets lost on its way to the table.

As host of a popular health show on a major New York City radio station (WMCA), I had the good fortune to spend time with Dr. Burkitt and other observant scientists during the early days of the fiber resurrection. Their insights taught me lessons not yet clarified in medical journals. I was also lucky enough to have opportunities to apply that knowledge, both personally and professionally.

My attention to fiber took a quantum leap with my first clinical experience. Here's the story: As a newly-appointed nutrition consultant at the Corsello Centers in Huntington, New York, I recommended a daily bowl of whole-grain cereal to Amy, who, at thirty-one, had been on medication for constipation relief more than half her life. Three weeks later, Amy returned to my office, smiling broadly.

ix

"It was so simple," she said. "Just a bowl of cereal. Why didn't anyone ever tell me about oatmeal before?"

Fiber advice is no longer based solely on hypotheses or clinical observation. Medical studies now offer compelling and clear evidence to explain *the consequences of fiber absent,* and *the benefits of fiber present.* The crucial importance of fiber is accepted as confirmed scientific and medical fact. Despite all the validation and current pageantry, however, ignorance abounds—especially when it comes to table talk.

Most of us recognize that there is no substitute for whole food. We all know that a natural food is more than the sum of its major nutrients. But (with deference to Amy), when it comes to fiber and the American foodways, *it's not always easy to consume a healthful, high-fiber diet on a daily basis!* And therein lies the problem.

Sure, you've been told that good health is yours for the picking. *But the pickings have to be conveniently available.* You may have the best intentions (especially on each New Year's Day). You resolve—year after year and many times in between—to lunch on a leafy-green salad, munch on an apple in the midafternoon, and crunch on a carrot during coffee break. But moments of reform are short-lived. Well-stocked veggie bins are not de rigeur office equipment. The Surgeon General's feel-good advice is *too little, too late; too often, too hard.* Shelf life and convenience belong to cookies and coke, not cucumbers and cauliflower.

BODY-CELL ANIMATION

We instinctively withdraw our hand when we touch something hot, just as we quickly jump out of the way of an oncoming vehicle. Wouldn't it be helpful if, when we consume highly processed foods, our body cells would withdraw or jump out of the way? Or perhaps our cells could emit video arcade noises and fireworks each time we allow corrupt food to slide down our gullet—after which we would go *TILT,* just like an over-manipulated pinball machine.

Can you imagine the colorful and noisy scenes in every restaurant and home kitchen serving high-fat, high-salt, high-sugar, overprocessed meals? In my dream, attention is focused on the root beginnings of the disease process. Our bodies would scream "NO" before damage was done. These warning signals couldn't be ignored! We would all take note if our tissues talked to us before it was too late—if we could *hear* and *feel* them breaking down.

A blender and quality fiber mix are also in my vision, mandated by federal law—side by side with the usual coffee dispensers that are already in place on every kitchen counter and in every office.

Tony, my seven-year-old grandson, summed it up succinctly: *"Grown-ups talk healthy, Grandma,"* he said, *"but they don't eat healthy."*

That's precisely why these chapters on fiber nutrition have been written.

Betty Kamen

Addendum:
Reflecting on the first edition, it is obvious that the conclusions presented continue to be validated again, and yet again—even as I edit the fourth edition. To demonstrate the point, here are a few additional studies published in prestigious medical journals as recently as the last few months:

Journal of the American Dietetic Association, June 1992. Dietary fiber is particularly low in away-from-home eating patterns among well-educated, higher-income women.[1]

Journal of Nutrition, June 1992. An inverse relationship is found between plasma cholesterol concentration and fecal excretion of bile acids.[2]

American Journal of Clinical Nutrition, June 1992. The importance of dietary fiber for insulin sensitivity has been confirmed. Low dietary fiber intake correlates with diminished insulin sensitivity in otherwise healthy lean and obese subjects.[3]

International Journal of Cancer, May 1992. Inverse associations with cholesterol levels are observed with dietary fiber. Such dietary factors may alter the risk of pancreatic cancer.[4]

Carcinogenesis, May 1992. Dietary fiber supplementation with pectin or guar gum (fed during the promotional stage of carcinogenesis), is found to suppress colon cancer incidence to a significant extent.[5]

Behavioral Medicine, Spring 1992. Hostility measures among women are negatively related to fiber intake.[6]

Magnesium Research, March 1992. Calcium supplementation inhibits magnesium absorption on a fiber-free diet, but has little effect on magnesium absorption when fiber is present. Absorption of calcium is increased by including some fiber in the diet.[7]

Indian Journal of Physiology and Pharmacology, January 1992. The overriding influence of physical form, cooking, processing, storage and antinutrient content of food is powerful. The lowest glycemic [blood sugar] responses occur when meals contain the largest number of nutrients.[8]

Nutrition and Cancer, 1992. A diet containing fiber affects the excretion pattern of a food carcinogen. There's a lower uptake and a decreased transit time through the gastrointestinal tract in a more diluted form than occurs with a nonfiber diet. Furthermore, less radioactivity is retained in the kidneys on a fiber diet.[9]

Nutrition and Cancer, 1992. Dietary fiber is believed to protect against colorectal cancer, and one of the ways it may act is by *adsorbing* mutagens that are carcinogenic.[10]

The trend is obvious. Even the FDA reopened its public comment period to reconsider its proposed rules regarding three health claims for diet/disease links. *These included dietary fiber and its correlation with cardiovascular disease!* The reopening is based on significant new studies provided to the FDA regarding the link.

BK

CHAPTER 1

FIBER
WHAT IT IS

The following caption jumped out at me as I scanned the week's medical journals:

APPLE JUICE IMPACTS ON BODY
DIFFERENTLY THAN WHOLE APPLE

And my brain froze in the moment of focus.

With ecstatic anticipation, I envisioned national headlines, blaring radio announcements, widespread coverage on TV talk shows. I was so elated, you would have thought I won the lottery. As it turned out, my naiveté was as over-blown as my excitement.

There were no headlines—not even a small blurb on a back page. *Nor was there a single response from the traditional medical community.* Of course, I should have known better. The year was 1977.

I wanted *everyone* to know about the value of fiber. But at that time, fiber meant nothing more to most people than threadlike strands woven into fabric. Writers used the word to describe character or strength. Nutrition science dismissed it as unimportant—a part of food having no nutritional merit, passing through your body unabsorbed. Today, however, fiber is having its time in the sun. The moment for fiber is NOW. At long last, the significance of the apple/apple juice study has gained recognition.

Why is fiber suddenly being touted as king of the good-health roost? (Even Johnny Carson referred to its importance recently.) The explanation is simple: Fiber is being removed from more and more plant foods, with catastrophic results. The correlations between fiber and disease are clear-cut, but reasons for the cause-and-effect/health-illness machinations are extremely complex.

Over and over, you've heard about the key operators of metabolism—carbohydrates, fats, and proteins. Referred to as macronutrients, their ratios vary from food to food. But each is almost always present in everything you eat. For example, even an apple contains low amounts of all the amino acids that make up the structure of human protein. *The full range of amino acids comprising human tissue is found in every single food.*

Surely you know that your bowl of breakfast cereal, your lunch sandwich, the fish you consume for dinner, are all reworked into you—sparking responses that convert to your strands of hair, to cells riding your bloodstream, to layers of your skin. Your food becomes the energy you use when you sit down to do your taxes, rush to answer the phone, or kiss your true love hello, good-bye, or good night.

The macronutrients (the carbohydrates, fats and proteins) have specific roles for helping food to become you—in keeping you alive and able to grow older—protected from agents of disease. Since fiber did not appear to have an active role in any of these processes, it was virtually ignored. Fiber was considered structural scaffolding, nothing more than the skeleton holding the peach or stalk of celery together; the part of the beet that gets discarded by your clever body because it has no biochemical use. Or so we thought.

Then it was noticed that Seventh-Day Adventists had lower rates of breast, colon, and other cancers than the general population. Several researchers suggested that this was because their vegetarian diet contained considerably more plant fiber. Mormons, although not vegetarians, also escaped the ravages of these diseases. Comparisons of the diets of traditional societies with those of industrialized communities began to flood the journals. Primitive groups, as noted by Denis Burkitt, were as free of the diseases of civilization as the Adventists and Mormons.

Subtle nutrition responses began to be recognized with more understanding, helping to crystallize Burkitt's observations. We made a mistake when we tried to explain food analytically. The molecular composition of fiber provided no insight into its powerful effects—until now. A food is, very definitely, more than the sum of its parts. Eating is a *total* phenomenon.

DEFINING FIBER

What is plant fiber and why has it kept certain populations free of diseases so common to other groups?

Dietary fiber is not a single substance. Lack of a clear definition of its consistency and differences in its various components mark its complexity. Since part of what we call fiber is not all fibrous, the very word is inaccurate.[1]

Fiber has been described as a series of different elements derived from cellular residues—stuff you cannot digest unless certain intestinal bacteria get a chance to work on some of these residues.

Denis Burkitt defined fiber this way:

> *Fiber is the part of food which is not digested. Whereas protein, fats and carbohydrates are almost entirely absorbed in the small intestine, fiber passes through to the large intestine virtually unchanged. Fiber does not provide energy or nutrients, or materials for growth and repair. It is the only component of our food that contains almost no calories.*[2]

We now know that components of some fibers *are* involved in metabolic responses during digestion. Kenneth Heaton, specialist in fiber-food experiments, added the following "spider-web" description:

> *Fiber of natural foods exists as a microscopic lattice-work or matrix which entangles and traps nutrients within cellular envelopes.*[3]

And here's a biochemical definition:

> *Fiber is a subclass of carbohydrates that consists of nonstarch or unavailable polysaccharides, its major constituents being cellulose, hemicellulose, lignin, and pectins which are not broken down into simple sugars during passage through most of the gastro-intestinal tract and are excreted in the stool.*

A ROSE BY ANY OTHER NAME

Regardless of title or definition, one thing is obvious: Dietary fiber can no longer be regarded as an inert filler. It is an integral ingredient whose role in your gut is a critical catalyst for health-promoting biological processes.

DESCRIPTIVE TERMS (For those who want to know)

Dietary fiber's reputation for reducing heart-disease risk and improving glucose (sugar) metabolism is now well established.[4] Associations of fiber deficiency with diseases such as appendicitis, breast cancer, colon and prostate cancer, colitis, diverticular disease, gastrointestinal disorders, gallstones, hemorrhoids, hiatus hernia, and ulcers have also been gaining acceptance. Fiber encourages health because it:
> ➤incorporates water
> ➤increases fecal bulk (a fact known since Hippocrates)
> ➤binds bile acids
> ➤reduces or normalizes total transit time
> ➤causes fermentation in the large bowel[5]

Explanations of these concepts relating to fiber, along with definitions of some general fiber categories, follow.

Bile Acids: *Acids formed in your liver and secreted in bile*
Eating a juicy cheeseburger? With French fries? Jambon à la crème? Ice cream for dessert? Not to worry. Bile acids to the rescue.

Bile is produced in your liver and stored in your gallbladder. Made from cholesterol (among other substances), bile acids are there to protect you after you eat a fatty or oily meal: They are called to arms to emulsify fats during digestion. After they mix with your fast-food lunch or gourmet dinner, the bile acids then take one of several trips. They go back to your liver or depart forever via feces.

Their selected itinerary could spell the difference between illness and health. (You might call this process the *ultimate acid test*.) In the presence of a significant percentage of fiber, bile acids take the exit route, and some of your cholesterol reserves are excreted rather than reabsorbed. If the bile acids go back upstream for want of fiber, you miss out on an opportunity to rid your blood of unwanted cholesterol.

Enzymes contained in bile acids also act as promoters of colonic tumors. Fiber dilutes the concentration of these evil mischief-makers by escorting them right out of your system. The process is called *bile-acid binding*.

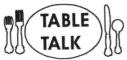 **TABLE TALK** Bile-acid binding is minimized when you swallow foods from which pectin has been removed. Consume the apple, not its juice.

In general, water-soluble fibers (found in oat bran, pectins from fruits and vegetables, and various gums found in nuts, seeds, and legumes such as beans, chickpeas, lentils, and peas) increase bile-acid excretion. Water-insoluble fibers (found in wheat bran and other whole grains, vegetables, and legumes) do not.[6] (See page 7 for definitions of soluble and insoluble fibers.) Each source of dietary fiber binds each of the bile acids with different degrees of efficiency. Remember that bile-acid binding is the desirable effect—that's what helps you to clear the bile acids, thereby keeping cholesterol levels stabilized and tumor incidence at bay.

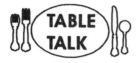 Hydrogenated and partially-hydrogenated foods inhibit the beneficial bile-acid-binding process. Check labels of peanut butter, margarine, salad dressings, baked products, nondairy whiteners, etc. You may be surprised at how many substances are hydrogenated. It is not in your best health interest to consume foods which inhibit bile-acid binding.

Bran: *The outer husk of any cereal grain*

Definitions are often settled by common consent and usage. Although not originally classified as dietary fiber, bran now "belongs," and is referred to as "cereal fiber." Most of the so-called, or now-called, dietary fiber of a grain is found in the seed's outer coat—the very part cast away in milling to make white flour.

Minimal breakdown of the outer layer of bran may occur during passage along the gastrointestinal tract. To the best of knowledge, the mass of bacteria in the cecum (the part of your large intestine where fermentation can take place) is unable to digest bran. Bran does, however, contribute to fecal bulk.

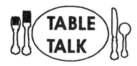 The fiber potential of cereal grain is in its outer coat, which is removed or mutilated in processing. Eat whole grains (millet, buckwheat, and brown rice are the best), rather than cold, boxed, over-refined "cereals."

Fecal bulk: *Stool volume*

Most types of fiber increase stool volume, and you can't help noticing this fecal volume change when you begin to increase fiber intake. Here is one "test" or observation that allows *you* to be the scientist. When noting this change, take inventory as to whether you're a "sinker" or a "floater." If you're a sinker, you may be headed for trouble. One caution, however: Poor fat digesters may also be floaters, even if they are not getting enough fiber.

Fermentation: *Partial breakdown of dietary fiber by bacteria*
The right side of your colon, or cecum, has been called a "fermenter." Fermentation converts poorly absorbed substances to more efficiently-assimilated matter.[7] The floral bacteria itself adds to fecal bulking and acts as a carrier to help get rid of unwanted substances. Fermentation assists in maintaining a normal, slightly acid pH level in the colon, crucial for intercepting colon cancer. (The pH level denotes acidity or alkalinity.) Dr. J. H. Cummings, reporting in *Lancet*, says, "Fermentation may be the single most important factor in the physiologic effects caused by fiber."[8]

Insoluble Fiber: *Fibers that do not dissolve in water*
Although most foods contain both soluble and insoluble fiber, one or the other type usually predominates. Examples of insoluble fibers are hemicellulose, cellulose, and lignin, found in whole grains and certain vegetables.

Soluble fiber: *Fibers which dissolve in water*
Soluble fibers are found in oat bran, apples, beans, and psyllium seed husks.

Total dietary fiber: *The sum of soluble and insoluble fibers*
Sixty grams of total dietary fiber is an average daily intake in developing countries. The National Cancer Institute has determined that America's daily intake ranges from a low 9.1 grams to a high of 13.8 grams. These figures were much less than expected.[9] The Institute suggests between 25 and 35 grams of fiber a day—for children as well as adults. The American Dietetic Association agrees. But many clinicians and research scientists recommend 50 grams daily for optimal health. No recommended dietary allowance has been established by the regulating agencies as yet.

> We consume very little whole-grain cereal, a bit more of the legumes, much more fruit, and a great deal more bread. Unfortunately, most of our bread is fiber-depleted.

Transit time: *The length of time it takes for pizza or potatoes—or anything else you eat—to travel through your system*
Transit time can be divided into segments, including gastric emptying, small-intestinal transit, and colonic transit. Gastric time is, however, ordinarily measured as the *total* intestinal transit time from beginning (your mouth) to end (your end).

Transit time averages only about one and a half days in rural communities in the Third World, but reports of seven- or eight-hour transits are not unusual. In Western countries, it's three days in young healthy adults, ten or more days among the constipated, and two weeks for the elderly. Even the range for each individual can be a great variable: A sweep from 47 to 123 hours in the same person is customary.[10] The only factor that reduces the fluctuation of your transit time is the addition of fiber to your diet, which, by reducing the time, appears to suppress the variation.

> The presence or absence of fiber is a major determining factor in your transit time. A high-fiber diet alters total transit by helping to normalize the action.

TRANSIT TIME

3 DAYS   10 DAYS   2 WEEKS

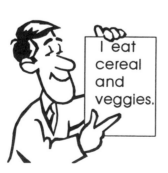

I eat cereal and veggies.

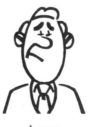

I am constipated.

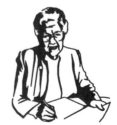

I am too soon old and too late smart.

The addition of fiber shows a more dramatic change in those with the slowest transit. Although fiber speeds the transit of the slowpoke, this may be reversed in those with too fast a transit. And so the concept of a normalizing role for fiber in gut action is demonstrated.[11] Substances which have this regulating effect are called *adaptogens*.

You can check your own transit time and once again have a chance to be the scientist. There are two ways to do this:

(1) Swallow a few kernels of raw corn (unchewed), and note how long it takes before the kernels appear in your stool.

(2) A more accurate method to determine transit time is with the use of charcoal tablets—the same tablets recommended for the treatment of intestinal gas, available at any drug store in 10-grain units. Between meals, swallow 5 to 10 tablets (with water), or whatever equals 20 grains or 1 gram. For the most authentic and precise result, take the tablets immediately after a bowel movement. Record the day and the time you start the process. When you first note the black, crumbly, charcoal-looking output, record the number of hours elapsed since you first swallowed the charcoal. You now know your transit time.

Remember that transit varies with your diet, so consume the foods you ordinarily eat for a few days before administering the test and continue until you get your transit result.

> The optimal transit time for healthy people is twelve to eighteen hours.

Was your transit time too rapid? Although possible, it is highly unlikely on a typical American diet. If, however, it was less than twelve hours, you may be depriving yourself of adequate time for digestion and food assimilation. You may want to consult a physician. A racy transit is *not* disadvantageous, however, as long as you are eating a high-fiber diet.

Too slow? That's more likely. The fortune cookie reads, "Danger ahead unless eating habits change. Add fiber to your diet." Correlations between specific disease conditions and slow transit are detailed in Chapter 3.

Why all the fuss about transit time? When it takes two to three times as long for your hard-working intestines to push its contents from your stomach to your anus, all sorts of interactions occur in the mass—*including the production of carcinogenic substances.* The longer the transit, the greater the possibility that putrefaction will lead to unhealthful waste products. Under certain circumstances these residues can even be reabsorbed from your colon into your blood stream and interfere with proper metabolism.

The quantity of fiber required is being standardized as that amount which produces a transit of not longer than three days, although this qualification is not yet official.[13]

Transit time is subject to great individual variation. Among the reasons for divergence:
~ degree of efficiency in food absorption
~ amount of cereal fiber consumed

Water-holding capacity: *Ability to hold water, like a sponge*
Good water-holding capacity of foods you ingest helps to ensure that your bowel content remains large in volume and soft in consistency. Increased fecal water content dilutes the concentration of a carcinogen in your body.

The different water-holding ability of food depends on:
➤the age of the plant
➤the amount of corruption (or processing) the plant has been subjected to—the further removed from its natural state, the less likely it is to mop up water
➤the quantity and quality of the plant's fiber makeup[14]

The preparation of fiber alters its water-holding capacity. For example, freezing, by compressing the fiber, makes the water unable to expand the plant's collapsed capillaries.

The point is that increased water content of the colon could dilute concentrations of carcinogenic compounds. How the food you consume affects this water-holding capacity is determined not only by *what* you eat, but also *how* that food has been stored and prepared.

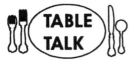 Baked potatoes have a greater water-holding capacity than potato chips; apples greater than apple sauce; and carrots greater than carrot juice.

FRUIT AND VEGETABLE FIBER COMPONENTS

Again and yet again we have heard how fruits and vegetables are good for us. We never questioned exactly why. Now we know.

The structural or matrix fibers of fruits and vegetables are lignins, cellulose, and some hemicelluloses. Their gel-forming fibers are pectins, gums, mucilages, and some hemicelluloses. More important than nomenclature is what these fibers do for us and how we can include them in our diets with ease. Among the benefits: cellulose and hemicellulose protect through effects on bowel contents; pectin and lignin protect through cholesterol-binding capability. Here are the specifics:

Cellulose: *Insoluble; the only truly fibrous component of the plant cell wall*

Cellulose is the best known, most widely distributed cell wall. An important property of cellulose is its ability to take up water and swell. This sponge-like characteristic of cellulose is the explanation for its ability to increase fecal weight. Although not yet totally definitive, there is a correlation between stool weight and freedom from disease, as cited above. This easily-discernible characteristic of waste matter is a telltale sign of health status.

Warning: Beware of confusing ingredient listings. The term *cellulose* suggests that a product contains important fiber. Right? Not always. Cellulose can be derived from many types of plants, including wood! *Cellulose added to some foods can be a wood pulp by-product.* Not enough studies have been done to determine whether or not wood pulp can be handled by the human digestive system. The suspicion is that sawdust does not react in a similar fashion to the cellulose found in edible plants, although it will reduce transit time.[15] When a high-fiber bread product was introduced in the United States in the 1970s, Canada refused to sell it because of its content of wood pulp. Canada's rejection of the bread created consumer awareness here, and now the amount of wood fiber allowed in our bread and any other product is limited, but still permitted. (The FDA decided it didn't want any isolated fiber replacing digestible grain products.)

Cellulose is listed on packaging as *methyl cellulose,* which may or may not be from an acceptable source. By contacting the manufacturer, I audit suspect products for their fiber derivation and quantity. I know from experience that the FDA does not have enough police power to inspect every manufactured product.

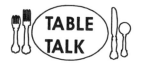

The best way to get a response from a manufacturer is to call or write the company, advising that you are deathly allergic to certain substances (such as wood pulp, if that's what you're investigating), and must have an ingredient disclosure.

Hemicellulose: *Forms the matrix of the plant cell wall (together with pectins) in which the cellulose fibers are enmeshed*
Hemicellulose is broken down by friendly microorganisms in the colon more readily than cellulose. This is a significant health benefit. Some types of hemicellulose, such as that found in psyllium husk, have a tremendous water-holding capacity.

Pectin: *Gel-forming substance contained in all fruits and many vegetables*

Pectin's ability to form gels is as important in human nutrition as in the jelly jar. If you have preserved jams and marmalades, you know all about pectin's use as a thickener. Prior to commercial availability of pectin in isolated form, your great-grandmother may have added apples to the jelly-making mix because of their pectin content. Pectin, for use as a nutritional supplement, is also derived from lemons, carrots, grapes, and several other fruits.

Pectin changes from an insoluble material in an unripe fruit to a much more water-soluble substance in a ripe fruit. (Didn't Mom tell you not to eat that pear or banana until it was ripe?) Again: soluble fibers are fermented to a much greater extent by colonic bacteria than insoluble fibers. Soluble pectins are almost completely fermented.

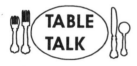 Processed foods are shorn of pectin. Obviously, this is not in your best health interest. If you consume an orange or strawberries in favor of orange juice or strawberry jam, you avoid the problem.

Gums: *A group of water-soluble or water-swellable fibers, or their derivatives*

Substances usually referred to as gums have also been used in foods for many years to impart such properties as thickening and gelation. Gums are only partly digestible, but provide water-binding and bulk to colonic contents. The presence of several gums in the diet has been shown to exert a significant cholesterol-lowering effect.

Gums are highly soluble, and are sometimes called *mucilages*. They are not part of the plant cell-wall structure, but are generally indigestible, so they are considered a component of dietary fiber. Locust bean and guar are examples of gums derived from seeds, as are agar-agar and carrageenan.

Lignin: *A highly complex molecule occurring in woody plant tissues*
Virtually indigestible, lignin has commercial value as a source of
vanillin and other aromatic chemicals.

Lignin is very inert and insoluble. The lignin content of the
fiber source affects the degree of breakdown of the fiber in your colon.
Its value is its ability to attract bile acids to its surface.

HOW FIBERS DIFFER

It is obvious that not all dietary fibers are created equal. Although
fibers have similar characteristics, their differences outweigh the
features they share.

Don't be concerned about all the details noted on the following
pages. The contrasts are offered only to indicate that distinctions
exist—an important concept in helping you to choose high-fiber foods
and/or a good fiber supplement (which is outlined for you in the last
chapter). No one should require post-graduate work in biochemistry
to figure out how to eat for optimal health and energy.

➤Fruits, vegetables, and grains contain varying amounts of soluble
and insoluble fiber. Example: Psyllium husk is about 90 percent
soluble; wheat bran is only 2 to 3 percent soluble.

Soluble fiber	Insoluble fiber
~ lowers cholesterol	~ aids digestion
~ reduces heart disease risk	~ aids elimination
~ improves blood sugar	~ promotes regularity
~ lowers blood pressure	~ contributes to bowel
~ promotes growth of friendly flora	cleansing

➤The more soluble the fiber, the more easily it is broken down, and
thus the nutrients in its complex structure are more usable. This quality
differs significantly with the fiber source.[16,17] Example: Wheat bran is
not as freely degraded as peas, carrots, cabbage, or apples.[18]

➤Different fiber sources have varying effects on intestinal transit. Examples: Pectin does not alter transit time; cereal fiber does.[19] Rice bran and wheat bran have similar accelerating effects on transit time.[20]

➤Cellulose is found in all plant cell walls in differing amounts. Example: Oats and barley are particularly rich sources; vegetable fibers have intermediate values.

➤Colonic bacteria does not affect all fibers to the same degree. Examples: Vegetable fibers stimulate colonic fermentation more effectively than do cereal brans.[21,22] Consistent intake of psyllium husk results in greater colonic microbial metabolism than intake of cellulose (as found in wheat bran).[23]

➤Different fibers have different stool-bulking abilities. Examples: Cereal fiber is a more effective stool-bulking agent than fruit or vegetable fibers.[24] Rice bran increases fecal mass and frequency of elimination more than wheat bran. Yet, as stated, both rice bran and wheat bran have similar accelerating effects on transit. Note these fiber effects on stool-bulking:

FIBER	STOOL-BULKING CAPACITY[25]
Bran	127%
Cabbage	69%
Carrot	59%
Apple	40%
Guar gum	20%

➤Laxative reactions appear to predominate with insoluble fibers. Example: Wheat bran has a greater laxative effect than guar.

➤Some fibers affect blood fat levels more than others. Examples: Wheat bran and soy bean fiber offer little change in blood fat levels, but pectin can lower cholesterol by up to 10 percent.[26,27]

➤Not all fibers contain the same amount of pentose. Pentose, a form of simple sugar, exerts the greatest influence in increasing stool bulk and softness—factors inversely related to cancer risk.[28] Examples: Cereal fiber is high in pentose; fruits and leaf vegetables are not.

FIBER ADDS BULK TO STOOLS BECAUSE:
- ~ it has terrific water-holding capacity
- ~ it has the ability to increase bacterial mass due to fermentation
- ~ it is poorly digested; most of the fiber is not broken down by enzymes, unlike other food components

---

➤Certain fibers change with maturation or cooking. Examples: Carrots, beets, radishes, and celery become increasingly "woody" with age, developing more cellulose. Overripe fruits form larger quantities of pectin. Heating reduces the glycemic advantage of guar gum.

➤Different fiber sources have different effects on mineral absorption. Examples: Beet fiber increases zinc and iron absorption. Wheat bran has no effect on iron, but reduces zinc. (The inhibitory effect of wheat bran may be due to its high phytate content, explained later.)[29]

➤Some fibers affect sugar metabolism. Examples: Sugar-beet fiber improves glucose tolerance; soybean does not. Soybean fiber enhances insulin levels; sugar-beet fiber does not.[30]

➤The water-holding capacity of fibers differ. Examples: Hemicellose has a greater water-holding ability than cellulose, but both adsorb more water than lignin. (*Adsorb* refers to gathering on the surface, rather than being incorporated, as in *absorb*.)

Are you confused? Wait! Please don't chuck it all and go back to your fast-food diet! All you really need to know is:

> Fiber is more than a simple substance
> The role of fiber in promoting health depends on its individual properties
> Fiber from different foods vary; e.g., fiber from an apple is different than fiber from wheat
> *You require a variety of fibers for optimal health*

WHERE FIBER IS FOUND

Foods are often compared in three and a half ounce amounts, or 100 grams—amounts equal to about the size of a fist. Note the very small quantity of fiber in 100 grams of apples, potatoes, and celery.

FOOD	QUANTITY OF FIBER in 100 grams
Apple	2 grams
Potato	2 grams
Celery	2 grams

Dr. Heaton, the physician experimenting with food fiber, explains that a 100-gram apple is, in a way, 98 grams of apple juice, held together by 2 grams of fiber. A similar amount of potato is about 98 grams of starchy mush, also held together by only 2 percent fiber. Despite the almost minuscule quantity, the fiber content, even if only 2 percent, confers a particular texture and architecture to the whole food—just as a small amount of emollient can alter the cohesion of a large batch of cream, or a small dose of yeast can make a large cake rise. So, although fruits and vegetables are composed mostly of water, they are solid.

> Fiber in an apple, even though present in minute quantities, is accountable for its firm consistency. Remove its modest amount of fiber, and you upset the apple cart. The same is true of every other plant food.

As an example of how significant the smallest measure of fiber may be, look at the differences in metabolism caused by equicaloric amounts of apple and apple juice—the results of the very experiment that suffused my world with joy in 1977:

(1) Insulin responses vary. Your insulin response to apple juice is 50 percent greater than that to whole apples.

(2) Satiety responses differ. You are hungry sooner after apple juice than after the whole apple.

(3) Transit time varies. Transit is more accelerated after eating the whole apple than after drinking its juice.

(4) Blood concentrations of cholesterol are modified. Apple juice raises cholesterol; whole apples help to lower high levels.

(5) A rebound fall in blood glucose follows consumption of apple juice, but not of whole apples. The high sugar content causes your blood glucose to shoot way up after you drink the juice. Because of all that sugar in your blood stream, your cells, which constantly communicate with each other, shout, "Hey, let's get rid of this excess sugar." So insulin springs into action to do the job. But *too much insulin* is excreted in response to the sugar oversupply, lowering your blood sugar beyond the point of normalcy—dropping it more than the value acceptable for optimal well-being. This rebound effect is much less likely to occur when you eat the whole apple. Sugar from apple juice enters your blood more quickly than it does from a whole apple, and that's what makes the difference.

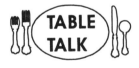 **TABLE TALK** Low blood glucose stimulates your appetite. Fruit juice contributes to overweight. Consume whole fruits, not fruit juices. Keep your blood sugar more stable.

Recall that in these experiments the amount of calories in a whole apple equals the amount of calories in the apple juice. So, comparing *apples to apple juice* can be a metaphor with the same connotation as *apples to oranges*! Different forms of the same food react like different foods because of the lack or presence of fiber.

FIBER FOODS: FROM HIGH TO LOW

(1) Highest quantity of fiber:
>Whole grain cereals
>>wheat, rice, corn, barley, rye, buckwheat, millet, oats

(2) A little less fiber:
>Legumes
>>peas, beans, lentils
>Nuts
>Seeds
>Dried fruits

(3) Still less fiber:
>Root vegetables
>>potatoes, carrots, parsnips, turnips, beets

(4) Even less fiber:
>Fruits
>Leafy vegetables
>>lettuce, cabbage, celery

(5) No fiber:
>Meat
>Chicken
>Fish
>Eggs
>Milk and milk products
>>cheese, yogurt, buttermilk

Bran, isolated from whole grains, leads the fiber pack; whole-grain cereals have more fiber than their cellulose-containing companions; *fruit is not exactly a high-fiber food*; and leafy greens, although teeming with other virtues, have the least amount of fiber in the garden patch. But the quantity of fiber in a food product appears to be less important than the frequency of consumption.[31]

The functions and values of fiber are determined by factors other than quantity.[32]

ALTERED FOOD

When whole-plant foods have been mushed, mashed, and mangled, the fiber is almost always left behind. Among the most extreme revisions have been the fiber-stripping that takes place in the production of white flour and sugar. Other foods running a close fiber-depleting detrimental second include processed white rice, corn flour, corn flakes and other so-called "cold" cereals, pearled barley, molasses, glucose, and maple syrups. Add fruit juices, wines, and even beer (which contains fiber-free maltose), and you can see how you would have to be on an unusual diet to be totally exempt from consuming processed, fiber-bankrupt foods. Heaton sums it up:

> *Sugar and other products of sugar refining, such as syrup and molasses, are such a familiar part of today's diet that it is difficult to remember how abnormal they are. The health disadvantages of sugar are attributable wholly or in part to the fact that sugar has been separated from fiber before it is marketed. By removing fiber from carbohydrate,* **civilized people have deprived their food-intake-controlling mechanism of one of its major cues.**[33] (Emphasis mine. More about fiber and appetite in Chapter 4.)

Removing fiber from food is like removing the weight-bearing walls of a house. The house slowly caves in on itself.

> We are artificially manipulating nature's own elaborate fiber-food design, and it isn't working.

It's hard to find fiber on an American menu.

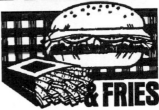

There's very little fiber here:

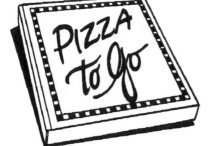

Or here!

And you know there's no fiber here:

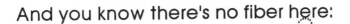

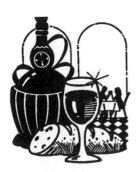

Or here!

FIBER IN FOODS

FOOD	SERVING	SOLUBLE FIBER (grams)	INSOLUBLE FIBER (grams)	TOTAL FIBER CONTENT (grams)
FRUITS				
apple	1	.84	1.96	2.80
banana	1 medium	.64	1.36	2.00
orange	1 small	.88	.88	1.20
pear	1 medium	1.00	4.00	6.00
raspberries	¾ cup	.37	6.43	6.80
BREAD				
white	1 slice	.25	.25	.50
whole wheat	1 slice	.25	1.15	1.40
CEREALS				
corn flakes	1 cup	.15	.25	.40
wheaties	1 cup	.47	2.13	2.60
RICE				
brown	½ cup	.20	2.20	2.40
white	½ cup	.01	.09	.10
VEGGIES				
asparagus	¾ cup	.81	2.29	3.10
broccoli	½ cup	.88	1.12	2.00
carrots	½ cup	1.11	1.19	2.30
lettuce	½ cup	.13	.17	.30
potato	½ medium	.95	.95	1.90
tomato	½ cup	.20	.60	.80
BEANS				
lima	½ cup	1.18	3.22	4.40
pinto	½ cup	2.02	3.28	5.30
kidney	½ cup	2.53	3.27	5.80

Note the high-fiber content of pears and raspberries, and the difference in total fiber content between brown rice and white rice.

More foods and their fiber content are listed in Appendix C, on pages 120 and 121.

CHAPTER 2

FIBER
WHAT IT DOES

No one can say my salad has everything in it but the kitchen sink. MY SALAD HAS EVERYTHING IN IT! My guests smile as they remove the small doll-house sink sitting atop their dinner salad. The message? Lettuce, tomato, and cucumber do *not* a salad make. *A salad is not a salad unless it contains at least ten different ingredients*—leafy greens, whole grains, grated raw tubers, the works—a kitchen-sink salad, with everything in it! Who counts? I do, and you should, too.

The reason for all this diversity? As discussed in the last chapter, *different fibers have distinct functions.* And you should have the advantage of each and every salubrious effect. Let's alter your insides for the better, or, better still, for the best.

> The characteristics of your intestinal contents are changed by the fiber sources in your diet.

It helps to think of fiber as a sponge passing along your gastrointestinal tract. Such a sponge has a water-holding and an exchange capacity. The sponge itself—the fiber—may pass through *unchanged* or *modified.* Either way, there are unique biological effects depending on the kind of fiber you consume. It has even been hypothesized that some components of fiber will function as antioxidants or free radical scavengers within your intestine.[1] (Antioxidants and free radical scavengers are highly protective molecules aimed at neutralizing toxins in your system.)

The following popular plant fibers are those you are likely to find in today's high-quality fiber supplement formulas. They are available in powder form, preferably in multi-mixes. Whether sold singly or in combo, you can purchase a large can and scoop out a measured quantity, buy a packet or bottle of capsules, or buy them tableted. You may even find some of these fiber sources added to formulas of vitamins, minerals, and herbs.

APPLE FIBER

Fruit fibers are becoming popular, probably because of their pectin content. (See page 37 for more on pectin.) Apple fiber initiates less of a blood-glucose response than the fiber of grapes, honeydews, oranges or strawberries.[2] Pectin is found to interact specifically with LDL-cholesterol, suggesting a biochemical basis by which it causes lower cholesterol levels.[3] A rather simplified explanation of LDL/HDL-cholesterol is that LDL (low density lipoprotein) is the "not-good" variety and HDL (high density lipoprotein) is the "good" stuff. The higher your LDL-cholesterol level, the higher the risk for atherosclerosis.

Test animals were fed diets to increase their cholesterol levels and then given a high amount of apple pectin. After two months, the apple product lowered the level of blood cholesterol. In the sixth month, cholesterol was depressed in the liver as well—by more than 50 percent.[4] The decrease was caused by reduced concentration of VLDL (very-low-density lipoproteins).

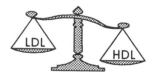

- Good: Heavy on the HDLs; light LDLs.
- Bad: Heavy on the LDLs; light HDLs.
- The ratio and balance between the two is the significant factor.

Insulin-dependent diabetics were given a milkshake and seven grams of apple pectin, equal to the amount in two apples, ten minutes before dinner. Following the meal, 35 percent less insulin was required to return blood sugar levels to baseline.[5]

How many times did your mother administer scraped apple when you complained of an upset stomach as a child? Part of the effectiveness of this remedy is attributed to pectin, which takes up water and provides bulk in a form that is soothing to irritated membranes. The soft absorptive mass helps harmful bacteria to escape—bacteria which might otherwise linger on your intestinal walls.

If the apple is organic, an apple a day, or its pectin-fiber equivalent, may indeed help to keep the doctor away.

BARLEY BRAN, BARLEY FIBER

Cereal grains and palm oil contain vitamin E (tocopherols) and *tocotrienols*. You may already be familiar with tocopherol as a lipid (fat) antioxidant, but the tocotrienols and their incredible functions have not yet received much press. (Watch for it!) Dr. Lester Packer, Ph.D., of the Department of Molecular and Cell Biology, University of California, Berkeley, has been focusing attention on this extraordinary substance. Packer says tocotrienols are many times superior to tocopherols in their role as antioxidants. When administered to test animals, these heavy-duty antioxidants increase lifespan, prevent platelet aggregation, and reduce cholesterol.[9] Platelet adhesiveness, or aggregation, refers to the clumping together of plate-like structures that appear in your blood which, when bunched up, restrict blood flow and contribute to heart disease.

Researchers at the University of Wisconsin have identified tocotrienols in the oil of barley bran. It has been known for some time that tocotrienols are found in the layers of cereal seeds,[10] and their isolation from barley bran is truly exciting. Tocotrienols have a definite cholesterol-lowering effect.[11] They give protection against certain types of experimental cancers in animals, showing promise for future use for humans.[12] Barley fiber also lowers cholesterol concentration in both serum and bile in test animals with gallstones. And it dissolves their previously formed gallstones.[13]

A recent study performed at the Division of Human Nutrition in Australia shows that barley fiber is more effective than wheat fiber in lowering blood cholesterol in men who have mildly high cholesterol levels.[14] Barley contains *beta-glucans*, a constituent of soluble fiber similar to that found in oat fiber, whereas wheat is comprised of the largely insoluble cellulose and hemicellulose fiber.

BEET FIBER

"Finish your beets!" is a phrase that may still strike an unpleasant chord in the hearts of many grown adults. We hear this command in our mother's uncompromising voice, and all the traumas and insecurities of our childhood are brought to the fore. No wonder. To the adolescent palate, the beet had to be the devil's vegetable.

But our mothers knew what they were doing. Without any formal nutrition education, they were aware that beets are one of the most remarkable (if often underrated) foods commonly found on the dinner plate.

One of the problems with beets is that they require a lot of cooking. Vitamin B_6 is critical to most of the beneficial actions of the nutrients in beets, but this vitamin is very sensitive to high temperatures. Since beets are usually boiled from thirty minutes to two hours at 212 degrees F, it's safe to say that a large portion of the original B_6 disappears in the process. Canned beets are subjected to even higher temperatures. We could eat the beets raw. But then we're back to measures that are out of kilter with late twentieth century lifestyle: convenience, lack of time for daily shopping, and so on.

Beet fiber has more soluble fiber than oat bran or rice bran, and very much more insoluble fiber than either.

The availability of beet fiber is new in the marketplace. Given the value of beets, it's no surprise that its fiber has been discovered to be beneficial. Beet fiber can:

➤help to normalize systolic blood pressure

➤decrease total cholesterol while increasing HDL-cholesterol, thereby lowering the LDL/HDL ratio

➤curb triglyceride levels[6]

➤improve glucose tolerance[7]

➤enhance iron and zinc absorption, important implications for mineral nutrition[8]

CARROT FIBER

Carrot fiber is a bile-acid binder. You already know the consequences: *It lowers cholesterol!* Six grams of carrot fiber (the equivalent of four or five small carrots) decreases cholesterol levels in those who need to lower these values.[15]

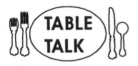 **TABLE TALK** Grate carrots into your salad. And/or keep carrot sticks handy at your desk or in your car. Transport and store in small insulated lunch bags or boxes. Use chemical ice to keep cold and crispy.

FLAX SEED FIBER

Essential fatty acids and *lignans*, the constituents of lignin, are bound up in flaxseed fiber. Lignans have antitumor, antioxidant, and anti-estrogenic activity. By binding estrogen, they lower cancer risk and help prevent tumor growth, as demonstrated in the chemotherapy program of the National Cancer Institute. Dr. Johanna Budwig of Germany reduces breast tumors with flaxseed oil and sulphur-containing protein foods. Flaxseed fiber contains naturally-occurring beta-carotene, B-vitamins, vitamins D_3 and E, plus an impressive assortment of amino acids.

GUAR GUM

Gums are a minor constituent in most foods. But certain gums have been used beneficially in isolated form, including guar gum, derived from the outer part of *Cyanopsis tetragonolobus*, a leguminous vegetable that grows in India. Guar prevents blood sugar from rising excessively after ingesting sweetened foods, so it is used as an adjunct in treating noninsulin-dependent diabetics. (Noninsulin-dependent, or late-onset diabetes, is referred to as Type II diabetes; juvenile or insulin-dependent, as Type I.) Guar also flattens glucose and insulin responses in normal people, and even in patients who have had gastric surgery.[16] Again—this means blood sugar does not climb as high as it normally would when ingesting sweetened foods if they are accompanied by guar. Presumably, guar, as with psyllium (described in a later section), accumulates water and forms gels in your intestinal tract, apparently delaying the absorption of the simple carbohydrates like sugar. *Guar moderates sugar absorption better than any other fiber.*

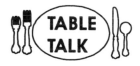 Consuming sweet foods, although not a recommendation for optimal health, produces fewer disturbances if accompanied by soluble fiber. Be sure to include a fiber supplement when eating sugar-laden foods.

Guar increases the excretion of fat by binding bile acids and fat.[17,18] (The same is true of pectin, to a lesser extent.) These results are considered by physicians and nutrition counselors in planning therapy when hyperlipidemia (elevated triglycerides or fat in the blood) accompanies Type II diabetes.[19]

And, like psyllium, guar is advocated for use in lowering total cholesterol when levels are too high. Clinical trials indicate that guar gum may reduce cholesterol by 10 to 15 percent.[20] The mechanism of action is thought to be similar to that of bile-acid binding and its capacity to reduce LDL.

Used with established cholesterol drug therapies (bezafibrate, lovastatin or gemfibrozil), guar gum may produce a further 10 percent reduction in total cholesterol. This is especially helpful for those who have not responded adequately to drugs alone.

The FDA is concerned about the use of guar gum as an isolated supplement. It is true that large, uncoated tablets of guar gum may cause problems. The tablet can swell prematurely, before reaching your stomach, and cause an obstruction. But guar gum has been shown to be absolutely safe in powder form, or when formulated with other ingredients—just the way you get it in a high-quality fiber complex. A recent article in the *Journal of Clinical Gastroenterology* describes guar gum as safe when used according to directions.[21]

Guar gum makes an excellent excipient and binder because of its texture and creaminess and because it does not "gum up."

GUM ARABIC

When certain plants are injured or exposed to adverse conditions, they exude a gummy material which dries in the form of lumps or ribbons. After collection and purification, the gum has many applications. In fact, it has been put to use for more than four thousand years.

Gum arabic is such a gum. Today, it is used in candy glazes, cough drops, lozenges, and as an addition to fiber supplements. A large percentage of ingested gum arabic may be assimilated and used for energy.

LOCUST BEAN GUM

Locust bean gum is an important gum, also used as a thickener and water-control agent in various foods. It is obtained from the seeds of the carob tree, an evergreen species indigenous to semi-arid areas of Spain, Italy, Greece, Cyprus, and Israel.

Locust bean gum is only slightly degraded during its trip through your gastrointestinal tract. Breakdown occurs by the microflora at the end of the line.

This fiber, like so many others, causes a decrease in total cholesterol due primarily to a decline in the LDL-cholesterol fraction.[22]

OAT BRAN, OAT BRAN FIBER

The oat-bran brouhaha has subsided. Advertising hype had us believing that oat bran alone was the cholesterol savior. Several other dietary fiber components (such as psyllium husk and guar) have been shown to reduce cholesterol levels about equally—facts known for some time, but only recently popularized.[23,24] Chapter 5 explains why it is not advisable to "settle" for a single fiber source.

Oat bran proved to ameliorate sugar-induced blood pressure elevations in hypertensive test animals.[25]

Oat *fiber* may be accompanied by a greater reduction in cholesterol than oat bran.[26] The cholesterol-lowering effect of oat fiber is associated with its soluble fiber content.[27] Oat fiber, which is extracted from oat bran, is more concentrated. Analysis shows that this greater concentration increases the amount of its soluble fiber content, so it is the more effective of the two for lowering cholesterol.[28]

WARNING: Some companies sell a product called oat fiber, which is made from oat *hulls*. These are high in fiber, but are insoluble, and will not lower elevated cholesterol. The product is relatively cheap and potentially deceptive.

PEA FIBER, PEA FLOUR

Years ago, when I baked and cooked (and was not yet a mostly-vegetarian), I added chickpea flour to bread recipes and mixed ground chickpeas into hamburger meat. Now I include chickpeas in my kitchen-sink salads.

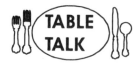 **TABLE TALK** Adding ground chickpeas (garbanzos) to hamburger meat will reduce the amount of meat (and its accompanying fat, hormones, and cost), and increase nutrient value. Garbanzos can also be added to mashed potatoes.

Fresh green peas became popular after a craze for them flourished at the court of King Louis XIV, when the passion for peas was described as "a fashion and a madness." Until then, they were eaten dried. Today, pea fiber is also a new kid on the fiber block. Peas are surprisingly high in fiber. Here's why pea fiber is beneficial:

➤Pea fiber has a cholesterol-lowering effect.[29]

➤Lysine, an essential amino acid often in short supply for vegetarians, increases with the amount of pea flour used.

➤The protein-efficiency ratio of your diet (or PER, a measure of the effectiveness of protein) is augmented by the addition of lysine.[30,31]

➤Pea fiber decreases blood glucose curves significantly.

Pea fiber is helpful for those who eat sweets as well as for diabetics because of its sugar-controlling effect.[32]

Egyptian research conducted years ago demonstrated that injecting pea extracts into the veins of dogs caused a temporary decrease in blood pressure.

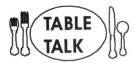 **TABLE TALK** Select a generous portion of chickpeas at the salad bar. Better still, sprout chickpeas and add them to your home-prepared salad or soups.

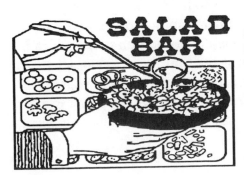

SALAD BAR

Soak dried chickpeas 48 hours, changing water in the AM and PM. Drain thoroughly; allow to sprout 24 hours in large jar or bowl, rinsing once or twice during that time. (Drain after each rinse.) Excellent nibble, just as is.

PSYLLIUM SEED HUSK

After millions of dollars spent on research and many years of experience, the American Heart Association recommended a heart-healthy diet beyond reproach. On such a diet, the experts told us, no other measures should be necessary. However, the diet lacked a sufficient amount of soluble fiber. The addition of psyllium husk enhances the cholesterol-lowering effect of the American Heart Association diet.[34]

The fate of LDL-cholesterol with the ingestion of psyllium seed husk:

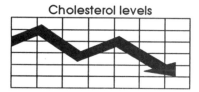

Cholesterol levels

Psyllium is easily tolerated by children as well as adults. It also spans the age groups in its ability to reduce total and LDL-cholesterol more effectively than the American Heart Association diet.[35]

In addition to moderating cholesterol levels, psyllium exerts a beneficial force on your glycemic index—your body's response to foods with sugar. Insulin levels are within a higher, but normal, range when psyllium accompanies your meal, indicating that it may delay the progression of diabetes.[36] Even if you are not threatened with diabetes, you can use this information to advantage. Eating pie à la mode sends your glucose soaring. Taking a psyllium supplement while enjoying your dessert helps to hold down glycemic responses.

Part of the reason for fiber's ability to tame your glycemic response is that it helps to delay the absorption of simple carbohydrates like sugar. By prolonging the time span over which the sugar is absorbed, psyllium even affects the metabolism of your next meal. The result is progressive with each successive meal, and so accounts for the long-term beneficial consequences of the fiber supplement.[37]

Slowly-absorbed foods prevent low blood sugar episodes, and psyllium is just such a food—it delays food absorption.[38]

Consistent intake of psyllium husk encourages good colonic microbial metabolism.[39] It stimulates the implantation and growth of the many strains of friendly bacterial cultures that make up the ecological system of your gut. Psyllium husk has the greatest bulking activity of the dietary fibers studied to date, making elimination smoother and more regular, and absorbing toxins on its journey through your system.

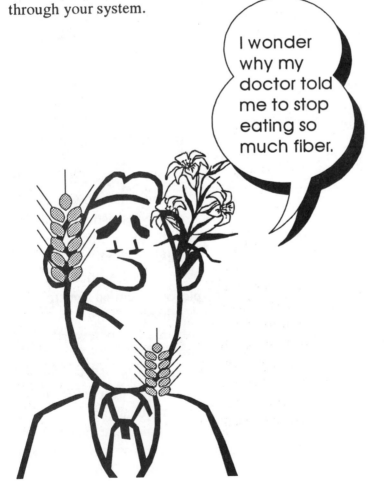

I wonder why my doctor told me to stop eating so much fiber.

RICE BRAN, RICE BRAN OIL, AND RICE FLOUR

It could be said that rice and humans have established a symbiotic relationship throughout much of the world.

Oryzanol, a substance found in the oil of rice bran, has unique implications for human nutrition. The biological name for rice is *Oryza sativa*, thus the name *oryzanol*. Even small doses of oryzanol enable certain cholesterol-controlling enzymes in your liver to function more effectively. Cholesterol levels of test animals maintained on rice-bran oil are significantly lower, with HDL-cholesterol higher. Oryzanol appears to contribute to the cholesterol-lowering ability of rice-bran oil.[40]

The protective properties of oryzanol go beyond that of simply lowering cholesterol. Oryzanol also reduces deposits of various other unwanted collections in your arteries.

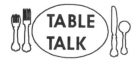 **TABLE TALK** White rice has no oryzanol. Ask for brown rice at the Chinese restaurant—repeatedly. If we all make the request frequently enough, it should become more available.

The study of oryzanol makes one wonder how a single substance can contain such an efficient mix of synergistic ingredients with such a wide range of protective contributions. It becomes less incredible when we realize that we're talking about a substance found in rice bran and that whole-grain, unprocessed rice has long since been the world's most popular staple food—culled from millennia of observant trial and error.[41] The dietary habits of survivors across the meshes of time have always been regarded as noteworthy and should continue to command our attention.

Rice bran as an isolated fiber, like other isolated fiber sources, is a new concept. Research investigating its effects on colonic function show that it increases fecal mass and stool frequency.[42]

Dieters, take note: It was also demonstrated that the combination of rice bran plus fish oil has a beneficial effect on fat metabolism. (This is not true of the blending of wheat bran and fish oil.[43])

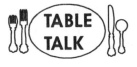 Prepare a brown rice side-dish with your fish meal instead of a baked potato. Order a fish dish in the Chinese restaurant if brown rice is available. (Push for that brown rice on the menu.)

In one significant study, ten patients with too much urinary calcium excretion were given rice bran for sixty days. The problem was reduced in all patients by an average of 40 percent, a very notable amount. Magnesium excretion was also lowered, and oxalate excretion increased.[44] My booklet, *Startling New Facts about Osteoporosis*, explains why these processes are effective for the prevention of osteoporosis. Is it possible that rice bran is an elixir for healthy bones? Is it possible that rice bran contains boron? Could the conversion from brown rice to bran-depleted white rice be a major cause for the increase of osteoporosis in Asian countries? What have we stumbled on here?

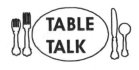 Add cold, cooked brown rice to your salads. It contributes so much delicious taste and texture, you'll find you won't require as much salad dressing. Salad dressings are depleted of fiber and are potentially rancid.

A formula based on high-protein rice flour was given to malnourished infants, and then evaluated. The acceptability, tolerance, and digestibility of most major nutrients were excellent. Some of the results proved to be equal to those of casein (milk protein). Weight gain was comparable to that attained with quality cow's milk-derived formulas in children of similar ages and nutritional status.[45]

Death associated with gallstones occurs when test animals are fed diets without fiber, but its incidence is eliminated by feeding the animals the same diet with rice flour plus fiber.[46]

Chinese people on traditional diets (including brown rice) have a low incidence of heart disease, with LDL-cholesterol levels far lower than levels found in Americans. How unfortunate that so much of the world has discarded the use of brown rice. How lucky that rice bran is added to exemplary fiber-food supplements.

SOY FIBER

Soybean-fiber supplementation significantly lowers total cholesterol.[47] It appears to counteract a high-fat diet by raising HDL-cholesterol levels. One study shows that a soybean diet actually reverses the progression of heart disease.[48]

Soybean fiber is also effective for reducing glucose levels in diabetics.[49] And it is among the few fiber types that will lower your triglyceride levels—which are normally raised after meals.[50]

WHEAT BRAN

As already noted, different cereal brans have distinct chemistries and water-holding capacities. Even the bran from the same cereal source may vary. Bran, for example, is different in hard, soft, or Durham wheat. The same applies to varieties of fruits and vegetables.

Every processing step changes the value of a food. The function of bran is altered by cooking, mixing, and pulverizing.

Bran in general reduces the number of tumors induced by chemical carcinogens.[51] Wheat bran may be effective in retarding colon cancer. The increased fecal weight and volume created by wheat-bran fiber appear to be involved in its inhibitory effect.[52] Wheat bran is shown to lower blood glucose and to increase the intestinal absorption of zinc.[53.]

Although wheat bran alone does not have important cholesterol-lowering effects, it drops cholesterol concentrations in diabetic patients by 30 percent when administered with guar gum.[54] No doubt there are many other synergistic effects at work that are still unknown—one more reason for *variety* in fiber and food selection.

Like so many other natural substances, wheat bran is also adaptogenic, operating only in the presence of need. In those with normal bile function, the addition of wheat bran has no effect on bile cholesterol.[55]

PECTIN

The fibers listed thus far are those derived from specific foods. Pectin is available from a wide range of fruits. (Commercial pectins, however, are produced almost entirely from citrus peel.)

Generally, pectin slows gastric-emptying time (the first phase of transit movement, when it is preferable for the food mass to move slowly). It improves glucose tolerance,[56] and may act through a mechanism similar to that of bile-acid binding in lowering plasma-cholesterol levels.[57]

Pectin reduces cholesterol concentrations an average of 13 percent. It increases fecal fat excretion by 44 percent and fecal bile acid excretion by 33 percent.[58]

Research was done to determine whether pectin has an immune-stimulating activity. The results suggest the possibility that pectin may act as just such an impetus.[59] Pectins are especially powerful in protecting against the toxic effects of some of the chemicals we consume with our food.[60] To the best of current knowledge, pectin supplementation has no adverse consequences on electrolyte (mineral) balance or glucose absorption.[61]

Among other fibers not detailed above are prune and fig fiber, popular because a small amount of the fruit contains large amounts of fiber.

Additional fibers found in today's formulas are xanthan gum, pear fiber, rye fiber, and even tofu fiber.

The fibers mentioned in this chapter are currently among those in popular use. The scenario, however, is not unlike buying computer equipment—before you bring your purchase home from the store, or before the amount due appears on your charge bill, there's an upgrade. The roster of fibers abstracted from original food sources is increasing rapidly.

As I write, a report is spewing out of my fax machine with information about *acerola fiber*. (Acerola is a type of cherry.) The analysis looks exciting—more lignin, more pectin, higher water-binding capacity, more of many other goodies than we find in psyllium-seed husk, guar gum, oat bran or wheat bran. Acerola fiber is now being incorporated into mixes produced by the health industry.

Will the tried and true have to jostle for prescription or appreciation with the newer fiber sources? Not necessarily. An important concept is that nature has many relay systems for health. And today's trend is for a potpourri, augmenting the classics with innovative fiber sources.

Fibers work best in combination, offering the advantages of the different fiber types.

SUMMARY

Whether new on the scene or tried and true, you now have an idea of why high-fiber supplements of quality are effective for maintaining health. Our advanced technology allows us to unfold nature's secrets as we weave fiber isolates, both new and old, into our nutritional regimen.

Physical properties of dietary fibers affect the functioning of the gastrointestinal tract and influence the rate and site of nutrient absorption.

Several physiological responses, such as lowering of plasma cholesterol levels, modification in the glycemic response, and improving large bowel function, have been associated with isolated fiber fractions or diets rich in fiber-containing foods.

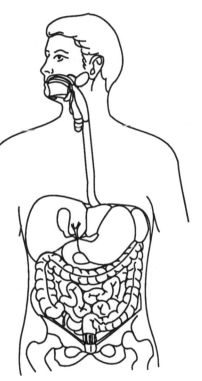

The Digestive System

Jane Brody, *New York Times* science editor, reported a fascinating account of the Indians of the American Southwest. Brody writes:

For the sake of their health, as well as their cultural heritage, the Pima and Tohono O'odham tribes of Arizona are being urged to rediscover the desert foods their people traditionally consumed until as recently as the 1940s.

....Preliminary studies have indicated that a change in the Indian diet back to the beans, corn, grains, greens and other low-fat, high-fiber plant foods that their ancestors depended upon can normalize blood sugar, suppress between-meal hunger and probably also foster weight loss.

These findings may also prove valuable to non-Indians who are susceptible to overweight and diabetes, and perhaps also those prone to high blood pressure and heart disease.

The benefits, which are also found in a few more familiar foods like oat bran and okra, stem primarily from two characteristics of the native foods: their high content of soluble fibers that form edible gels, gums and mucilages, and a type of starch called amylose that is digested very slowly.

The effect is to prevent wide swings in blood sugar, slow down the digestive process and delay the return of hunger.

....Even those Indians who still rely heavily on beans and corn are today consuming varieties that have little or none of the nutritive advantages found in the staples of their historic diet.

For example, the sweet corn familiar to Americans contains rapidly digested starches and sugars, which raise sugar levels in the blood, while the hominy-type corn of the traditional Indian diet has little sugar and mostly starch that is slowly digested.

San Francisco Chronicle, June 2, 1991, p. 2

CHAPTER 3

FIBER
HOW IT AFFECTS DISEASE

Perhaps Santa can spiral through your fireplace, but most adults cannot—not even in the long ago, when fireplaces were bigger. It was common practice in England to send young boys slithering through chimneys to remove soot. Over a century ago, an astute physician, Sir Percival Pott, noticed that many of his elderly patients with skin disease had been chimney sweeps as young boys. Although he knew nothing about cancer metabolism or the powerful carcinogens in soot, the physician related the condition to the job. He concluded it was the skin contact with the soot-impregnated clothes that caused the problem.

Time and again, medical history demonstrates causative associations between afflictions and particular factors in the environment. This can happen long before we comprehend the ways in which a specific disease may come about.

We are still groping for the *fiber-protection* answers—still searching for more precise explanations about how fiber works for relief or prevention of myriad abnormal conditions. Even as I write, a researcher on the radio is reporting a widely publicized new study on the association between breast cancer and lack of fiber. He is saying, "Fiber, *by some magical means that we don't understand*, is creating changes." (Italics mine. More about this research in the following pages.)

Just as you benefit from the power of electricity without full comprehension of how it works, you can profit from the incredible correlations between health and a high-fiber diet, despite a lack of understanding of the pathways involved. Increasing evidence of the roles of poor nutritional choices as a cause of illness are finally being emphasized in medical journals.[1] The bad news is that with the exception of lung cancer, the total cancer incidence in the United States has risen 27 percent since 1950, and the number of cancer cases is predicted to double by the year 2000 when cancer jumps to the number-one position for mortality.[2]

Evidence relating lack of fiber intake to ill health is overwhelming. After my exposure to Denis Burkitt's theories, it was years later when an astute friend, Larry Jordan, pointed out the relationship between breast cancer and fiber intake. Larry, a nutrition educator, has rare insight and is somewhat of a walking encyclopedia when it comes to medicine. It was no surprise to find medical validation for Larry's breast-cancer/fiber link. This led me to extensive research of other disease states associated with the absence of fiber.

In chronic diseases, a genetic condition may exist on which environmental variables work. Both factors interact. The propensity to a particular disease may be inherited, but whether or not that disease surfaces very often depends on your environment.

You can counteract heredity.

Let's look at the liaisons between fiber and common diseases—correlations associating prevention, intervention, and post-illness strategies.

The diseases and conditions explored are listed alphabetically; the studies cited for each grouping are in reverse chronological order. Detailed data are randomly scattered throughout the citations for the sake of interest. In most cases, only the conclusions of the studies are reported. This is by no means a complete list of fiber-related health problems, nor of the studies suggesting the ties.

APPENDICITIS

Definition
Inflammation of the appendix, a tube about two inches long, opening into the beginning of the large intestine.

Causes
Appendicitis is usually caused by a blockage from a small hard lump of fecal matter, which exists in the presence of the firmer feces associated with fiber-depleted diets. Under these conditions, unfriendly bacteria swarm into the appendix, resulting in inflammation.

Background information
Dr. Burkitt taught his Ugandan doctors to be wary about diagnosing appendicitis in an African—unless the African could speak English. Only an English-speaking African would have had exposure to Western ways, an association that could alter the African's lifestyle. Appendicitis still remains uncommon among communities having minimal contact with Western society. It is one of the first of several diseases, including colon cancer, that emerges only after transitions in lifestyle. This information and its tie-in with reduced dietary fiber has been recorded in medical journals for more than fifty years.

Mortality from appendicitis is negligible and morbidity slight. But appendectomy patients are at greater than average risk for certain cancers.[3] It may be that the fiber-depleted diet resulting in appendicitis is the same diet that sets the scene for cancer.

Appendicitis is a condition that is preventable and need never happen in the first place.

Culture comparisons are not the only benchmarks for the appendicitis/fiber connection: When food in British prisons was coarser than food eaten outside, appendicitis was less common among prisoners than in the rest of the population.[4]

Medical Validation: The Fiber/Appendicitis Connection

➤*Gastroenterology*, 1990. The increase in appendicitis is promoted primarily by an associated fall in dietary-fiber intake.[5]

➤*Cancer Research*, 1990. A link between appendicitis and large bowel cancer has been noted, and both are hypothesized to be prevented by a high-fiber diet.[6]

➤*British Journal of Hospital Medicine*, 1985. Since early in this century consumption of a low-fiber diet has been implicated in appendicitis.[7]

Putting the appendicitis puzzle pieces together is easy when you read the literature. One researcher reported that appendicitis arrived in his region in China in 1940 when a

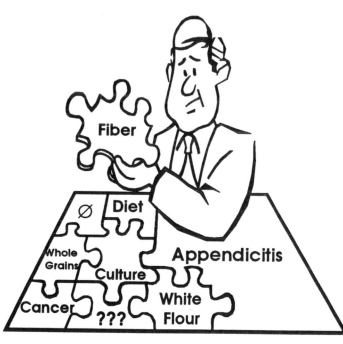

roller mill was installed. This is the machine that removes the bran and germ from the grain of wheat. Eventually, all cases of appendicitis occurred in government employees and in students eating flour from the roller mill. But the Chinese who were faithful to their traditional diet and continued to eat stone-ground flour remained free of the disease. It is interesting to note that none of the Chinese had access to sugar, so it appears that the lack of fiber in their cereal foods caused the problem.

BREAST CANCER

Definition
New growth of unregulated, abnormal cells in the breast. Cells continue to reproduce until they form a mass known as a tumor. Such tumors interrupt body functions. Untreated, they spread to other parts of the body and can be fatal.

Causes
Environment, heredity, and biological factors—including elevated estrogen—all play a role. The environmental factors, including diet, are now believed to be the most significant cause—particularly high intake of certain polyunsaturated fatty acids and a poor intake of antioxidants.

Background information
In a study published in April 1991 in the *Journal of the National Cancer Institute*, it was reported that laboratory test animals fed high-fiber diets developed fewer breast tumors than those receiving little or no fiber. This is the breast-cancer research I referred to at the beginning of this chapter—the study receiving widespread publicity. Leonard Cohen, M.D., at the American Health Foundation in Valhalla, New York, where the study was conducted, said:

> *We found that by doubling the amount of fiber in a diet that is similar to our Western diet, you can significantly reduce the amount of mammary cancer, down to the level of a low-fat diet. It shows that the fiber itself contains substances which, when they get into the bloodstream, will inhibit the formation of a mammary tumor. What seems to be happening is that fiber by some magical means that we don't understand is creating changes in the hormone system which protect against breast cancer.*

The release of this research created the sensation I had expected in 1977 with the publication of the apple/apple juice report. *The breast-cancer story became front page news and a major topic for talk shows.* A direct association with a specific disease and the current breast-cancer epidemic served as catalysts. According to statistics published in 1991 in *Preventive Medicine*, breast-cancer incidence rates in the United States have been climbing for the last 40 years, but recent trends have shown a more dramatic increase since 1982. The disease afflicts at least one in nine women—occurring in epidemic proportions, and affecting even more lives than AIDS.

> The number of women whose years are tragically cut short by breast cancer is still on the rise.

The American Health Foundation report is not the first study to link fiber deficiency and breast cancer. Nor do the theories all relate to the "magic" to which Dr. Cohen alludes. In 1986 an article entitled "Hypothesis: A New Look at Dietary Fiber," published in *Human Nutrition: Clinical Nutrition,* noted that breast cancer may be estrogen-dependent, and that dietary fiber increases the excretion of excess estrogen.[8]

In 1987, an interesting report was cited in the *Journal of Steroid Biochemistry*, advising that fiber intake causes the production of substances that protect against breast and prostate cancer.[9] The highest values of these substances (lignans, equol, and enterolactone) are found in those who consume macrobiotic, lactovegetarian, and traditional Japanese diets. These groups have a low risk for the development of breast and other hormone-dependent cancers. Japanese women have a small incidence of breast cancer until they move to the United States and adopt our fiber-depleted Standard American Diet, for which the appropriate acronym is SAD. (See the updated report of this research on page 47.)

Larry Jordan was ahead of his time. It was the fiber-hormone-cancer connection that he had already explained to me.

Medical Validation: The Fiber/Breast Cancer Connection

➤*Mutation Research,* 1991. Insoluble fiber, composed of hemicellulose, is a component that could remove certain mutagens.[10]

➤*Scandinavian Journal of Clinical and Laboratory Investigation.* Suppl, 1990. The results of a ten-year study show that diet is a significant or even the main factor increasing the incidence and mortality of breast cancer. A Western-type diet elevates levels of sex hormones. This increases undesirable steroids and results in decreased formation of mammalian lignans and other compounds— substances which could protect against cancer-cell growth. The precursors of these saviors are found in fiber-rich, unrefined grain products, various seeds, beans, and probably also in peas, lentils, and berries.

> Fiber influences sex-hormone and bile-acid metabolism mainly by increasing fecal excretion of the negative compounds.[11]

➤*International Journal of Cancer,* 1990. A high intake of cereal products, especially those rich in fiber, may be inversely related to the incidence of breast cancer.[12]

➤*Medical Oncology and Tumor Pharmacotherapy,* 1990. The approach to breast-cancer prevention should include an increase in fiber consumption to 25 or 30 grams a day.[13]

➤*Nutrition and Cancer,* 1990. Dietary fiber has the potential for affecting breast-cancer risk. Fiber may have a protective role because of its influence on estrogen metabolism and excretion, or because of the effects of good-guy lignans—a family of compounds formed in the intestine from fiber-associated precursors.[14]

➤*American Journal of Epidemiology,* 1989. Increased fiber intake is associated with a reduction in the extent of tumor densities, as shown on mammograms.[15]

➤*Journal of Steroid Biochemistry,* 1989. One study shows that only one single parameter separated premenopausal breast-cancer patients from two control groups, including both omnivores and lactovegetarians: *grain fiber!*[17]

➤*Journal of the National Cancer Institute*, 1989. The dietary patterns of the Western world (high-fat, low carbohydrates, low fiber) affect certain factors in breast cancer, such as tumor size and estrogen-receptor content of the tumor.[18]

➤*Cancer Research*, 1989. Fiber from grains consumed during early teen-age years results in decreasing the chances of breast cancer in both premenopausal and postmenopausal women.[19]

➤*American Journal of Clinical Nutrition*, 1989. A Western-type diet in postmenopausal women is associated with breast cancer.[20]

➤*American Journal of Epidemiology*, 1988. There are no indications that fat intake promotes breast cancer.[21] (This study assumes that the fat intake comes from whole, natural foods, rather than highly-processed rancid fats, a major component of our Western diet.)

More on breast cancer

In 1990, the *British Journal of Obstetrics* reported an increase in breast cancer risk since the first use of hormone replacement therapy. The longer the therapy is prescribed, the greater the hazard. Women with breast cancer represent the highest percentage of patients in the field of gynecological oncology. An extensive study in Germany shows that 70 percent of cancer operations are performed on patients with breast cancer. In March of 1991, the United States journal *Archives of Surgery* confirmed that the prognosis of inflammatory breast cancer has been poor. (Patients with cancer show an increased risk of committing suicide and the forms of cancer which most frequently involve suicide include breast cancer.)

Although I am citing the most recent studies, these associations have been known for many years. Can you begin to understand my excitement when I read the comparison reports of the effects of apple and apple juice fifteen years ago?

CANDIDA

Definition
Yeast-like fungus, normally part of the flora of the mouth, skin, intestinal tract, and vagina; can cause a variety of infections.

Causes
Friend or foe—antibiotics kill both with equal vengeance. While they destroy the bacteria causing your strep throat or other infections, they also wipe out healthful digestive organisms. When protective microflora are suppressed, the Candida cells multiply. In addition to antibiotics, Candida yeast overgrowth is also stimulated by birth control pills, cortisone and other drugs, and diets rich in sugar.

Background information
Candida bacteria are heavy players in human illness—more so than previously suspected. Both immediate and delayed sensitivity reactions to Candida are very common. According to William Crook, M.D., known for his work on the subject, any of these symptoms may be caused by Candida:

> headache, fatigue, depression, irritability, digestive disorders, respiratory disorders, joint pains, skin rashes, menstrual disorders, loss of sex drive, recurrent bladder and vaginal infections, sensitivity to chemical odors and additives.

There is also increasing evidence that gut yeast may be involved in some cases of psoriasis.[22]

Medical Validation: The Fiber/Candida Connection
➤*Journal of Family Practice*, 1989. The association between dietary intake and the history of vaginal Candida was evaluated in an extensive, controlled study. Among the results: There is an association between fiber intake and Candida. Outcome was not altered by controlling for age, body-mass index, smoking, use of oral contraceptives, and sexual-activity variables. In other words, even those women whose environments were conducive to producing Candida were able to be Candida-free with adequate fiber intake![23]

CHOLESTEROL (ELEVATED)

Definition

Fat-like substance required as a precursor for many important body processes, including cell-membrane integrity, nervous system function, and the production of sex hormones. Too much cholesterol is a misplaced or aberrant consequence of metabolism-gone-wrong, and can lead to gallstones and life-threatening deposits in arterial linings. These deposits are commonly found in the arteries of patients with high blood pressure, those who suffer sudden, very painful heart attacks, and patients who have had a stroke.

Causes

High levels of cholesterol are related to PROCESSED fats, and to stress. Nutrient deficiencies and a sedentary lifestyle have also been implicated. Indicting eggs and other whole, natural, *intact* foods which contain cholesterol has never been proved to be a factor.

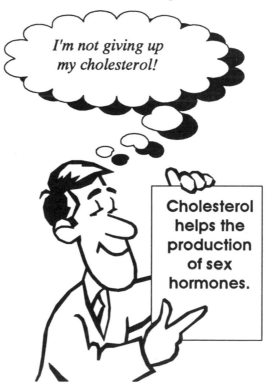

Background information

High levels of cholesterol in your bloodstream have little to do with consumption of whole foods, including eggs—even if they contain cholesterol. (Send a self-addressed, stamped envelope to Nutrition Encounter, Box 2736, Novato, CA 94948 for my white paper listing studies validating the fact that eggs do not cause raised cholesterol levels.)

> The real fear with regard to cholesterol should be that somehow someone hasn't told you the full story.

Physicians with a commitment to providing the best care for their patients have voiced concerns over the popularization of inaccurate cholesterol-testing programs. To complicate matters, some experts are anxious about the fact that many physicians prescribe drugs as treatments far too quickly. These drugs are expensive and potentially dangerous. Other less invasive methods often work to normalize cholesterol levels.

As stated earlier, high-fiber diets result in bile-acid excretion, thereby reducing the amount returning to your liver. To compensate, your liver produces more primary bile acids, using the cholesterol in your blood as part of the necessary raw materials, thereby pruning your cholesterol pool. If no additional cholesterol is manufactured, your cholesterol levels decrease.[24]

Medical Validation: The Fiber/Cholesterol Connection

➤*Journal of Gerontology*, 1991. Intake of fiber is inversely associated with total cholesterol levels in older people. The effect of dietary factors on cholesterol levels is not age-limited: elderly people may benefit from diet alterations.[25]

➤*American Journal of Public Health*, 1991. Daily inclusion of two ounces of oats appears to facilitate the reduction of total cholesterol in individuals whose levels are high.[26]

➤*AmericanJournalofClinicalNutrition*, 1990. Soluble-fiber cereals are an effective and well-tolerated part of a prudent diet in the treatment of mildly- to moderately-high levels of cholesterol.[27]

➤*Archives of Internal Medicine*, 1990. Psyllium in a twice-daily regimen may be a useful and safe adjunct to a good diet in the treatment of moderately-high cholesterol.[28]

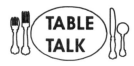 **TABLE TALK** Add a tablespoon of mixed soluble fibers (psyllium seed husk, guar, beet fiber, etc.) to your bowl of breakfast cereal.

➤*Proceedings of the Society for Experimental Biology and Medicine*, 1990. Propionate is a salt produced by bacterial fermentation of soluble fiber in your colon. This substance may inhibit cholesterol and fatty acid production and may be partly responsible for the cholesterol-lowering effects of soluble dietary fiber.[29]

➤*Journal of Atherosclerosis*, 1990. Cholesterol levels are reduced in those with high cholesterol by 9.6 percent with the intake of guar.[30]

➤*Journal of Clinical Pharmacology*, 1990. Psyllium (the active ingredient in Metamucil, sold for many years as a bulk laxative), can lower total and LDL-cholesterol and raise HDL-cholesterol. Psyllium is well-tolerated with long-term use.[31] Many people have switched from sugar-filled Metamucil to psyllium seed husk, available in natural-food stores.

➤*Journal of Nutrition*, 1989. When guar gum is the source of dietary fiber, dietary fats may not affect cholesterol levels.[32]

➤*The Journal of the American Medical Association*, 1988. Usually the last to admit that diet is preferable to drugs, JAMA made this statement:

> *A broad public health approach to lowered cholesterol levels by additional dietary modification, **such as with soluble fiber**, may be preferred to a medically oriented campaign that focuses on drug therapy.*[33] (Emphasis mine.)

➤*Journal of the American College of Nutrition*, 1987. Pectin, guar gum, and oat bran (soluble fibers) have been reported to have cholesterol-lowering effects proportional to the degree of cholesterol elevation. Other gums also lower cholesterol, with the decrease in total cholesterol due primarily to lowered LDL.[34]

> The higher or more abnormal your cholesterol level, the greater the percentage of reduction with the use of soluble fibers.

➤*Journal of Cardiology*, 1987. Bean fiber can decrease total cholesterol by as much as 19 percent, and LDL by 22 percent. Psyllium can reduce total cholesterol by 15 percent.[35]
➤*Proceedings of the Society of Experimental Biology and Medicine*, 1971. Psyllium prevents the accumulation of cholesterol. An increase in bile-acid excretion rates has also been reported.[36]
➤*Nutrition*, 1965. Pectin reduces cholesterol in test animals.[37]

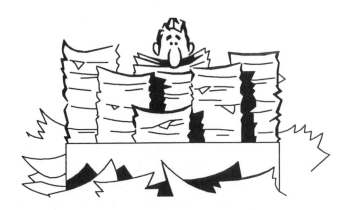

Voluminous medical literature validates the fact that dangerous cholesterol levels can be lowered with certain kinds of fiber.

COLITIS

Definition
Inflammation of the colon.

Causes
Colitis is caused by unwise eating habits; overdosing on laxatives.

Background information
"It's psychological. Go home and relax." Nothing can cause more stress than hearing these words from your physician. Everyone—especially the professionals—should know that telling someone to "just relax" simply does not work.

Because spasms occur in the early phase of colitis, it was believed that tension was the sole cause. There is no doubt that psychological factors can have an effect on body functions. But if your body is well nourished, stress-controlling mechanisms don't break down. Needless to say, the kind of optimal nourishment that prevents this kind of body breakdown is hard to come by.

Medical Validation: The Fiber/Colitis Connection
➤*Southern Medical Journal*, 1991. Two cases of colitis were resolved with psyllium therapy.[38]
➤*Digestion*, 1989. A fiber-poor diet is a major factor as a very high risk for the recurrence of colitis.[39]

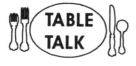

BARLEY WITH NUTS
Ingredients: 1 cup barley; 1 tbsp oil or butter; 2 cups vegetable stock; ½ cup chopped almonds.
• Brown barley in oil or butter; add stock. Cook over low heat, covered, until tender, about 1 hour. Stir in nuts, cover pan again. Simmer 5 minutes more.

COLON AND COLORECTAL CANCER
(also referred to as large-bowel cancer)

Definition
Cancer affecting the colon or both the colon and rectum. The large intestine or large bowel includes the colon and rectum. (Most of the large intestine consists of the colon, but the last six inches or so is the rectum.)

Causes
Low-fiber diets are associated with bowel cancer. Bacteria in the colon act on bile salts to create carcinogens.

Background information
Does it upset you as much as it does me to learn that, (1) colon cancer is our second most common type of cancer, (2) it is a major cause of mortality in the United States,[40] and, (3) the real tragedy: researchers acknowledge that patients need not die of colorectal cancer?[41]

Colon cancer is nonexistent in rural Africa, but both black and white Americans are at comparable risk—a striking example of its increasing prevalence associated with cultural change. The rates of colon cancer in various countries are inversely associated with the consumption of fiber—the more fiber, the less colon cancer.[42] Tumors of the colon are universally rare in Third World countries.

Mutagens (substances causing mutation of, or alterations to, natural structures), which indicate an increased risk of colon cancer, are found in the waste matter of individuals who consume the typical high-fat, low-fiber Western diet. Studies with newborns show that these concentrations appear early in life, but are not present at birth.[43]

Bile acids are the number-one culprit in this disease. In experimental studies, their damage to DNA, among other types of destruction, is largely prevented when the bile acids are pretreated with fiber.[44] If carcinogens leave your bowel quickly, they pose less risk, an event that occurs when they are diluted with large fecal volume. This is accomplished with a high-fiber diet. Fiber dilutes bacterial activity, thereby reducing the cancer potential.

Dr. Jerome DeCosse, of the Memorial-Sloan Kettering Cancer Center, confirmed that cereal fiber can act very rapidly to slow down colon cancer, even after initial signs have been diagnosed.

Consumption of a coarse rye bread popular in Finland has resulted in that country's fecal bulk being three times that of most Westernized nations. In addition, there was demonstration of a significant reduction in fecal bile-acid concentration. The incidence of colon cancer was reported to be less than one-third that of the United States, despite fat intake in Finland ranking among the highest in the world.[45] (Their incidence of coronary heart disease is another matter.)

Copenhagen Danes have four times the colon cancer risk of rural Finns. Both groups have similar fat intakes, but the Finns consume 80 percent more fiber. The same applies to comparisons between New Yorkers and Finns. It appears that the protective influence of cereal fiber may outweigh the deleterious influence of high-fat consumption.[46,47]

Assuming that the reduction of fat has the same health benefits as increasing fiber, increasing fiber is much easier to implement. (See Chapter 5.)

Medical Validation: The Fiber/Colon Cancer Connection

➤*Southern Medical Journal*, 1990. Increasing the intake of dietary fiber greatly decreases mortality associated with colorectal cancer.[48]

➤*Proceedings of the Nutrition Society*, 1990. Fiber-containing foods are protective in colorectal cancer. The effect is largely due to vegetable fiber.[49]

➤*Reviews of Infectious Diseases*, 1990. The activity of intestinal microflora and cancer of the large bowel are related. Enzyme-initiated cancer-causing substances can spring to action as a result of unfriendly intestinal bacteria. The levels of harmful colonic bacterial enzymes are inhibited by dietary fibers.[50]

➤*Tidsskrift for den Norske Laegeforening*, 1990. Poor dietary habits are associated with increased frequency of cancer in the large bowel. A low-fiber, high-fat diet increases the risk of developing a colonic neoplasm (any new, abnormal, uncontrolled growth).[51]

➤*Journal of the National Cancer Institute*, 1989. Dietary grain fiber and total dietary fat act as competing variables in the beginning stages of large-bowel cancer. The more fiber, the greater the health advantage.[52]

➤*Cancer Research*, 1990. Fat has no effect on cancer development when the fiber content of the diet is high. These results indicate that both dietary fiber and fat affect colon carcinogenesis in a complex, interactive manner.[53]

➤*Medical Oncology and Tumor Pharmacotherapy*, 1990. Despite a two and a half-fold increase in fat intake, there has been only a small increase in breast-cancer rates in Japan since World War II, . That fact and the lack of correlation between fat intake and risk of breast-cancer mortality among rural Chinese populations suggest that a major association between meat and animal-fat intake and risk of breast cancer is unlikely or weak.

➤*Anticancer Research*, 1989. Dietary iron may augment colorectal cancer risk. One of the mechanisms by which fiber diminishes colorectal cancer risk may be the chelating, or "grabbing" of dietary iron by the phytic-acid component of the fiber.[54]

➤*American Journal of Epidemiology*, 1989. Dietary fiber decreases colon cancer risk.[55]

➤*Nutrition and Cancer*, 1987. The effect of using psyllium husk (water-soluble) and cellulose (water-insoluble) against chemically-induced colon cancer was investigated in test animals. Animals were fed similar diets, but one group was fed psyllium husk and the other cellulose. Tumors were induced in one-half of the animals fed each diet. Psyllium strongly reduces the tumorigenicity (tendency to cause tumors); cellulose has a more moderate effect. The psyllium diet also increases fecal output, while the cellulose regimen tends to result in greater fecal bulk.[56]

CONSTIPATION

Definition
Slow movement of very firm content through the large bowel leading to infrequent passing of small hard stools.

Causes
Constipation represents a common social phenomenon today, associated with modern habits of diet and lifestyle. Many studies show lack of fiber and insufficient water intake as causes of constipation.[57,58]

Background information
Imagine a serious and debilitating ailment that afflicts one in fifty people in the United States at a cost of more than $300 million a year. Imagine the Nobel Prize bestowed on the scientist demonstrating a cure for that condition. Imagine what we could do with $300 million saved! Well, my friends, it doesn't take imagination, money, or award-winning scientists. Constipation, one of the most chronic digestive disorders in the United States, can be eliminated (pun intended) overnight.

High-fiber foods provide moisture-retaining bulk so that waste matter in your colon won't become dry and tightly packed.

Water and other fluids have no effect on constipation without fiber. In the absence of fiber, fluid is simply absorbed from the bowel and excreted in urine.

Medical Validation: The Fiber/Constipation Connection
➢*Journal of Gerontological Nursing*, 1990. The supplement of dietary fiber reduces hunger and increases the frequency of elimination.[59]
➢*Postgraduate Medicine*, 1990. A simple, helpful measure for chronic constipation includes dietary-fiber supplementation.[60]

➤*Orthopedic Nursing,* 1990. Patients hospitalized for surgery or confined to bed are at high risk for constipation. Patients who eat more fiber request fewer laxatives.[61]

> Soy fiber improves bowel function even in a nonambulatory population, a group usually suffering from bowel disorders.[62]

➤*Minerva Dietologica E Gastroenterologica,* 1989. It is necessary to introduce fiber into the everyday diet to be able to prevent or cure constipation.[63]

➤*Minerva Pediatrica,* 1989. Vegetable fibers represent an effective treatment of functional chronic constipation in children.[64]

➤*Journal of the American Dietetic Association,* 1987. The most consistent benefit of consumption of adequate dietary fiber is regular elimination. Conclusion of the study: "This effect alone justifies inclusion of fiber in the diet, in view of the enormous expenditure on drugs for digestive diseases."[65]

➤*Scandinavian Journal of Gastroenterology,* 1979. Bran is significantly superior to a bulk laxative for constipation.[66]

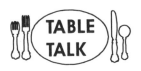

TABLE TALK

CONSTIPATION COMMENTARY
Delete: over-refined foods; hard-boiled eggs; cheese; meat; boiled milk; hot drinks; foods containing tannin (tea, cocoa, red wine); cloves.
Add: foods that absorb moisture readily (celery, radishes, carrots, lettuce); foods that are slightly laxative (raw figs, raw spinach, strawberries, sesame seeds, watermelon); garlic (prescribed for constipation by Hippocrates); agar-agar, taken with lots of water; dandelion leaf tea; flax seeds; brewer's yeast; rice polishings; and the herb *cascara sagrada*.

CORONARY HEART DISEASE

Definition
Condition existing when arteries supplying blood to your heart are narrowed by plaques compounded from oxidized cholesterol, calcium, fats and proteins.

Causes
You've heard the warnings time and again. Smoking is the strongest risk factor. You are also in jeopardy for heart disease when you are under stress, eat the wrong foods, live life in the fast lane, don't get adequate sleep, and do not exercise.

Background information
Coronary heart disease is our number-one killer and a major public health problem. Too many Americans die annually from cardiovascular disease—tragedies that need not occur. The American Heart Association diet lowers cholesterol in a limited number of people.

Many individuals, including professionals, have been led to believe that cutting back on fat or cholesterol is the sole key to heart health. In a widely publicized article that appeared in the *New England Journal of Medicine* in 1977, George Mann, M.D., said, "The emphasis on fat has kept preventive cardiology at a standstill for the past twenty years."[67]

> High cholesterol is NOT the most significant factor in coronary heart disease.

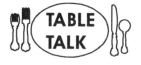

Although smoking is the mighty peril, and processed fat is a well-documented heart hazard, cereal fiber can be a Herculean heart helper. Heart health could be as simple as eating a bowl of oatmeal, millet, or brown rice every day.

Medical Validation: The Fiber/Coronary Heart Disease Connection

➤*American Journal of Clinical Nutrition*, 1990. Dietary fiber lowers blood fat and blood pressure.[68]

➤*American Journal of Cardiology*, 1987. Soluble fiber decreases estimated risk for coronary heart disease by greater than 30 percent.[69]

➤*Atherosclerosis*, 1987. Soy fiber was studied alone and in combination with soy protein. The results suggest a complementary role for soy fiber and soy protein in preventing atherosclerosis.[70]

➤*New England Journal of Medicine*, 1986. In a study of a thousand men of Irish descent, those who died of coronary heart disease had lower intakes of dietary fiber.[71]

➤*New England Journal of Medicine*, 1985. Two years on vegetarian diets protected thirty-nine coronary heart patients from further lesions.[72]

➤*Lancet*, 1982. There is an inverse correlation between dietary fiber intake and coronary heart disease. Fewer than five percent of men in the highest third for cereal fiber intake develop coronary heart disease.[73]

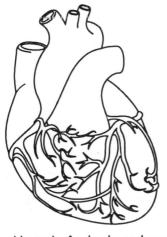

Soluble fiber decreases estimated risk for coronary heart disease by greater than 30 percent.

Heart; Anterior view

DENTAL CARIES

Definition
A destructive process causing decalcification of tooth enamel, leading to cavities.

Causes
Causes of tooth decay are not completely understood, but some facts are known. Like other degenerative diseases, this is also a disease of civilization attributed to refined foods, which translates to lack of fiber.

Background information
Sucrose is among the highest cavity-causing substances. Although there is no simple relationship between food sucrose content and caries,[74] the fact that foods with refined sugar lack fiber is obvious.

Medical Validation: The Caries/Fiber Connection
➤*British Dental Journal,* 1990. The severity of the processing undergone by snack foods and the nature of the flavoring (i.e., sugar) determine the cariogenic effect. More processing equals more cavity-causing. More processing, less fiber. For example, salted peanuts are not as cavity-producing as cheese-filled puffs. Some varieties of cheese and onion snacks may cause as many cavities as semi-sweet biscuits.[75]

➤*Leber, Magen, Darm,* 1988. A higher intake of dietary fiber is important in the prevention of caries. A mixture of several kinds of fiber with water-binding and bile-acid binding capacity is preferable.[76]

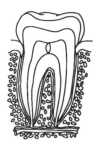
You only get
one set. Take
care of it.
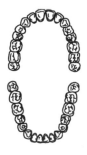

DIABETES

Definition

Any disorder characterized by excessive urine excretion and decreased carbohydrate tolerance. Blood sugar rises too high and then appears in the urine. Diabetes mellitus is a disorder in which the ability to use carbohydrates is impaired because of disturbances in normal insulin mechanisms, causing glucose to be denied entrance to the cells.

Causes

The disease is most likely to occur among those who eat refined, low-fiber carbohydrate foods.

Background information

Ah, to be a hunter-food gatherer, such as an African bushman or a Laplander. Among the advantages, you would be assured of remaining free of diabetes. Diabetes takes an enormous human and monetary toll each year. Current treatment often revolves around insulin and drug therapy. According to James Anderson, M.D., diabetologist at the University of Kentucky, fiber can reduce insulin requirements, improve glycemic control, lower cholesterol and triglyceride values, and promote weight loss in diabetics. We have known for more than a decade that a high-fiber diet leads to discontinuance of insulin therapy in about 60 percent of noninsulin-dependent diabetics, and significantly reduces doses in the other 40 percent.[77]

> ~ For diabetics, short-term use of fiber lowers blood glucose and insulin requirements.
> ~ Long-term use of fiber lessens the likelihood of specific complications of the disease.

In Japan, India, and the West Indies, where the intake of carbohydrate and dietary fiber is high, the specific complications of diabetes are less frequent.[78] Within one or two decades after changing from a high-fiber to a low-fiber diet, Yemenite Jews and the Transvaal Bantus have shown an increase in the prevalence of this sugar-disordered disease.[79]

"Fiber can ultimately improve metabolic control and decrease health-care costs," says Anderson.[80]

Many types of dietary fiber modulate glucose absorption. The outcome: reduced levels of glucose and insulin following meals. This effect may be due in part to delayed gastric emptying in the presence of fiber.[81] Water-soluble fibers are much more effective in lowering glycemia than insoluble fibers.[82]

The terms *insulin resistance* and *insulin sensitivity* should be understood for clarification of metabolic pathways.

Insulin resistance refers to cells which are insensitive to insulin. It's as though the cells put up a "DO NOT ENTER" sign. As a result, too much insulin remains in your blood, and many processes are thrown out of whack. An over-supply of insulin sets you up for fatigue, stress, overweight, and heart disease.[83]

Insulin resistance can be caused by a deficiency of biologically active GTF-chromium (glucose tolerance factor). Chromium is an essential trace mineral. According to Richard Anderson of the United States Department of Agriculture, chromium deficiency is rampant—more than 95 percent of Americans are chromium deficient! Why? You know the answer by now. Chromium goes down the drain when foods are processed—it is found in greatest amounts in the hulls and coarse outer portions of grains.

Because of the extensive problems generated by chromium deficiency, niacin-bound chromium is a popular supplement. Chromium is also found in high amounts in brewer's yeast.

Recent research shows great promise for *vanadyl sulfate* as beneficial treatment for diabetes. Vanadyl sulfate is the safe form of the mineral *vanadium*.

Insulin sensitivity refers to the ability of your tissue to open the doors to receive insulin, which is just what you want. Insulin is the key to getting glucose into your cells.

> Too much insulin increases unnecessary manufacture of cholesterol. It affects your energy level, stress-coping abilities, weight-control mechanisms, and even your muscle and fitness potential.

Medical Validation: The Fiber/Diabetes Connection

➤*American Journal of Clinical Nutrition*, 1990. Dietary fiber improves glucose metabolism.[84]

➤*American Journal of Clinical Nutrition*, 1990. High-carbohydrate, high-fiber diets increase insulin sensitivity in healthy people—young and old.[85]

➤*Journal of the Association of Physicians of India*, 1990. Two and a half hours after ingestion of glucose, platelet adhesiveness rises significantly in diabetics as compared with normal individuals. After a glucose load taken with fiber, platelet adhesiveness falls significantly. Fiber supplements may prevent or delay the vascular complications usually associated with diabetes.[86]

➤*International Journal of Clinical Pharmacology, Therapy, and Toxicology*, 1990. Guar gum improves metabolism and decreases serum lipids in patients with noninsulin-dependent diabetes.[87]

➤*Revista Clinica Espanola*, 1990. Accumulated experience suggests that an increase in carbohydrate intake (60 percent of the diet), most of which should be fiber-rich, is recommended—given its proved efficacy in better control of blood sugar and lipids. Such a diet is of major importance in noninsulin-dependent diabetes.[88]

➤*British Journal of Nutrition*, 1990. Supplementation with soluble fiber improves glucose tolerance.[89]

➤*American Journal of Clinical Nutrition*, 1989. Retinopathy, a disease of the retina, is a common manifestation among diabetics. Patients without retinopathy have significantly higher daily intakes of total fiber than patients who develop retinopathy.[90]

➤*Diabetes Educator*, 1989. Soluble dietary fibers are associated with health benefits for diabetics. A flexible approach for inclusion of dietary fiber in diabetics is recommended.[91]

➤*Journal of Internal Medicine*, 1989. Adding appropriate wheat bran to the diabetic diet is helpful for diabetic control and the correction of zinc deficiency.

➤*American Journal of Clinical Nutrition*, 1988. Sustained pectin ingestion slows the gastric-emptying rate and improves glucose tolerance.[92]

➤*Annals of Nutrition and Metabolism*, 1988. Sugar levels rise more slowly after a meal made with guar-gum spaghetti. Glucose levels at one hour after the guar-gum spaghetti meal are roughly equal to the glucose levels at thirty minutes after the meal with ordinary spaghetti.[93]

➤*Indian Journal of Physiology and Pharmacology*, 1988. A significant fall in blood sugar is exhibited with intake of psyllium.[94]

➤*Journal of Clinical Nutrition*, 1987. Obese Type II diabetics were fed a standard meal with or without 10 grams of soy fiber, enhancing the return of glucose levels, and reducing the rise of triglycerides.[95]

➤*Clinical Science*, 1984. Soluble fiber improves glucose tolerance, flattening the blood-glucose response.[96] This occurs because of slow absorption—the kind achieved on high-complex carbohydrate diets.[97] Among the many fibers studied, guar was most effective in delaying transit time (by seventy-five minutes!).[98] Because of the delay, slow absorption and improved digestion take place with the next meal consumed, even if the next meal is devoid of fiber.

With a high-fiber diet, diabetics may eventually decrease their insulin dosage or tablet medication.[99]

➤*American Journal of Clinical Nutrition*, 1976. When diabetic patients on low doses of insulin are treated with high-carbohydrate, high-fiber diets, insulin requirements are reduced.[100]

➤*Lancet*, 1977. The addition of guar gum to the diet reduces the amount of sugar in urine, regardless of insulin dose.[101]

DIVERTICULAR DISEASE

Definition

Development of small, blown-out, or inflamed pouches in the wall of the colon, usually manifested as pain of abrupt onset in the lower left quadrant. Complications may occur with or without an acute attack.

Causes

Increased pressure on the bowel wall because of the additional physical effort required to propel firm feces causes diverticular disease. This form of mechanical damage, only recently investigated, is considered a key factor in the development of this disease.

A low-fiber diet produces maladaptive changes in the colon resulting in high pressures. Too little fiber messes up the action of the bowel. One indication of this is the formation of diverticuli, the blown-out pouches. As with so many other processes, the tensile strength (or stretching ability) and elasticity of your colon decline with age.[102]

Background information

After departing from traditional eating habits, it takes a culture about forty years to develop a high prevalence of diverticular disease. But it doesn't take that long to put a stop to its progression. Mortality in Britain from diverticular disease came to a screeching halt in 1940. Fiber intake had risen to nearly forty grams a day as a result of World War II processed-food restrictions.[103] With the exception of war constraints, this disease is closely related to economic development. The more prosperity, the more diverticular disease.

The disease is consistently found more frequently in omnivores, or in those vegetarians who have a lower intake of cereal fiber. Unfortunately, vegetarianism doesn't always mean healthful eating habits. I have one vegetarian friend who subsists on doughnuts for breakfast, white-bread sandwiches for lunch, and pizza for dinner. Many vegetarians are really *meat-avoiders*—nothing more.

The role of high-fiber diets in reducing bowel-wall pressure is primary.

Some people with diverticular disease may be asymptomatic, while others experience pain and bowel disturbance along with additional symptoms. Complications include infection, bowel obstruction, and bleeding. The disease may be life-threatening and is called a deficiency disease of Western civilization for good reason, having become increasingly more common in industrialized countries during this century.

Medical Validation: The Fiber/Diverticular Connection

➤*British Journal of Clinical Practice*, 1990. A high-fiber diet is effective in the treatment of diverticular disease.[104]

➤*Surgical Clinics of North America*, 1988. Colonic diverticulosis is truly a disease of the late 1990s. A direct correlation exists between the incidence of diverticular disease and the amount of dietary fiber.[105]

➤*Primary Care; Clinics in Office Practice*, 1988. Diets low in fiber predispose a patient to the development of diverticulosis, and adding fiber to the diet is effective in prevention and treatment.[106]

➤*Medical Aspects of Dietary Fiber*, 1980. Fiber of cereal origin appears to be the most important component of dietary fiber for protection against diverticular disease. (Whole grain cereals, of course—not the boxed shelf-life "cereal" pretenders.)[107]

➤*Clinical Gastroenterology*, 1975. Early in their development, diverticula, like other hernias, are reducible. Dietary fiber is the antidote.[108]

➤*American Journal of Surgery*, 1973. Low-residue diets have never been proved to arrest the development of diverticula or to prevent complications. In fact, evidence shows that such diets cause symptoms to persist.[109]

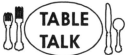

Kind-To-Your-Stomach Recipes
1. Dried prunes soaked overnight in water with lemon juice.
2. A blend of 1 tbsp pumpkin seeds, 2 ounces of sesame seeds, 1 cup of soaked raisins. Add enough warm water to make one quart. Sip through the day.

SUMMARY: DIVERTICULAR DISEASE

~Those on low-fiber diets are more prone to develop diverticular disease.

~Low-fiber diets produce maladaptive changes similar to those seen in diverticular disease.

~When treated with high-fiber diets, patients with diverticular disease experience symptom relief.

~On high-fiber diets, the high pressures within the colon are reduced.

~An association between diverticular disease and varicose veins, hiatus hernia, and hemorrhoids has been reported.

~Those people with the greatest inherent weakness of the bowel wall develop diverticular disease most readily, and at a younger age.[110,111]

GALLSTONES

Definition

Stonelike masses that form in the gallbladder. The gallbladder is a sac that stores bile for the digestion of fatty foods.

Causes

The more cholesterol in your bile, the greater the tendency for gallstones to develop. Gallstones cause trouble by blocking the duct between the gallbladder and the main bile channel, or by blocking the main channel itself.

Background information

When your gallbladder acts up, gallstones are usually present.

Removal of the gallbladder is one of the most frequently-performed abdominal operations.

Fiber increases the production of a substance which helps keep bile cholesterol in solution. The use of fiber to improve bile composition followed the observation that rural Africans rarely form cholesterol gallstones.[112] If you have normal bile composition, fiber has no effect. Again, the adaptogenic paradigm—fiber works only when needed.

Gallstones are most common in women after pregnancy, in obese individuals, and in men and women past thirty-five. In Western populations, about one-third of elderly women have gallstones—an incidence that increased during this century.

Medical Validation: The Fiber/Gallstone Connection

➤*Lipids*, 1990. The highest incidence of gallstones is found in animals receiving the lowest fiber diets. Gallstone incidence is reduced by dietary fiber.[113]

➢*Apmis*, 1990. Barley fiber reduces cholesterol concentration in both serum and bile in test animals with gallstones. It also dissolves previously-formed gallstones.[114]

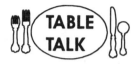

Barley-Soy Waffles
Ingredients: 2¼ cups water; 1½ cups whole barley, 1 tbsp oil; 1 cup soaked soybeans (½ cup dry). • Soak soybeans and barley several hours. Drain; discard water. Combine all, and blend until light and foamy, about ½ minute. Let stand while iron heats. Batter thickens on standing. Bake in hot waffle iron 8 minutes. Can be baked ahead. Soaked beans and barley can be kept in fridge for a week, at the ready.

➢*Journal of Nutrition*, 1989. Death in test animals is associated with gallstones when the animals are fed diets without fiber, but the incidence of gallstones is essentially eliminated by rice flour plus fiber.[115]

➢*American Journal of Gastroenterology*, 1989. In South Africa, the incidence of gallstones is reported to be increasing in urban blacks. Their recent dietary changes include a rise in fat consumption and a fall in intake of dietary fiber.[116]

➢*Canadian Journal of Surgery*, 1978. After four weeks, nine patients demonstrated a significant decrease in bile cholesterol simply by adding bran to their regular diet. Three of the patients continued on the diet for another six months and showed an increase in HDL-cholesterol.[117]

➢*Z Erna*, 1975. Lignin reduces cholesterol gallstones in test animals.[118]

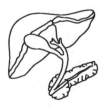

The gallbladder is a pear-shaped organ. Here you see the gallbladder and the pancreas and spleen. The gallbladder is attached to the under-surface of the liver.

HEMORRHOIDS

Definition
Swollen anal cushions, pushed down through the anal canal.

Causes
The passage of hard feces forces anal cushions down, leading to hemorrhoids. Constipation is a fundamental underlying cause.

Background information
Like so many other diseases of civilization, hemorrhoids are common in Western countries, and rare in the Third World. (Has this been sounding like a broken record?) The passage of small, firm stools has been implicated in hemorrhoids. High-fiber stools, being soft and pliable, are readily molded and propelled by the colon, and decrease transit time.

Medical Validation: The Fiber/Hemorrhoid Connection
➤*Acta Chirurgica Scandinavica*, 1988. A high-fiber diet increases the long-term cure rate among patients with third-degree hemorrhoids. The number of treatments required for cure of hemorrhoids is lower when bran is added to the diet.[119]

➤*Diseases of the Colon and Rectum*, 1987. Postoperative hemorrhoid patients receiving fiber have shorter hospital stays and suffer less pain. In general, all-around recovery is accelerated and fewer side effects are experienced.[120]

➤*Human Nutrition: Applied Nutrition*, 1985. Fiber improves stool bulk and intestinal transit time to encourage the healing of hemorrhoids.[121]

➤*American Journal of Gastroenterology*, 1984. Bulk-forming fiber supplements are a first-line therapy for hemorrhoids.[122]

> On-going fiber-depleted diets can cause hemorrhoidal conditions so severe that prolapse of the anus occurs—a falling down or slipping out of position. (Cosmetic surgery has no place in anorectal disease.)

HIATUS HERNIA

Definition
A condition in which the top of the stomach is pushed upwards out of the abdomen and into the thoracic cavity, the part of the body above the diaphragm.

Causes
Straining to pass small firm stools is a major cause.

Background information
Although hiatus hernia frequently occurs without symptoms, some people experience heartburn because of the entry of gastric acid up into the gullet. Hiatus hernia is among the diseases that are rare in traditional societies consuming high-fiber foods.

Medical Validation: The Fiber/Hiatus Hernia Connection
➤*Lancet,* 1985. A low-fiber diet increases the risk for hiatus hernia.[123]
➤*Lancet,* 1973. Unnaturally raised intra-abdominal pressures necessary to evacuate firm stools resulting from consumption of low-fiber diets are an important factor.[124]
➤Any study illustrating the use of fiber to avoid straining is applicable here. Review the research cited under CONSTIPATION.

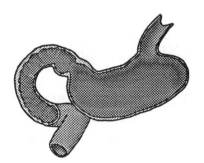

Your stomach does
a yeoman's job.
Treat it kindly.

HYPERTENSION and STROKE

Definition
Persistently-high pressure of blood against arterial walls.

Causes
Hardening of the arteries is one cause. Fluid buildup due to sodium retention or mineral imbalance, such as potassium deficiency, may be significant. (Refer to my book, *Everything You Always Wanted to Know About Potassium But Were Too Tired to Ask.*) Additional precursors are obesity, smoking, hyperactive personality, and stress. It may also be the result of other disease states, such as adrenal tumors.

Background information
Don't you know at least several people on high-blood-pressure medication?

> More Americans will die this year from circulatory disorders than in all our wars combined.[125]

   Vegetarian groups consistently maintain lower blood pressures than matched control groups. Fiber helps to keep your circulatory system unobstructed.

Medical Validation: The Fiber/Hypertension, Stroke Connection

➤*Postgraduate Medical Journal*, 1990. Multiple dietary intervention (in this case in the form of a low-sodium, low-fat, *high-fiber* diet), is more effective than any single dietary treatment and is useful in patients already on high-blood-pressure medication.[126]

➤*American Journal of Gastroenterology*, 1986. A study comparing high-fiber diets with liquid diets in twenty obese subjects showed that the high-fiber diet was more effective in decreasing high blood pressure.[127]

➤*Nutrition Research*, 1985. Three hundred health-food shop customers received an increased cereal-fiber intake of 100 grams a week. Reduction in both systolic and diastolic blood pressure followed.[128]

➤*British Medical Journal*, 1979. A comparison of fiber intake and blood pressure in 94 healthy individuals revealed that those with high-fiber diets have significantly lower blood pressure than those with lower fiber intakes.[129]

➤*British Medical Journal*, 1979. A group of seventeen healthy volunteers was asked to increase fiber intake modestly by making high-fiber substitutions for low-fiber foods. Blood pressure dropped significantly over a four-week period.[130]

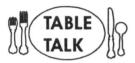

TABLE TALK

ORIENTAL BROWN RICE
(My favorite high-fiber, low-fat inexpensive meal-in-a-dish)

Ingredients: 1 cup brown rice; 2½ cups water; 4 tbsp sesame oil; 2 cups bean sprouts; 1 cup green peas; 1 cup chopped scallions; 1 cup diced water chestnuts; 1 cup mushrooms; 1 cup chopped celery; 1 cup chopped green or red peppers; 4 cloves mashed garlic; 3 tbsp tamari; 2 eggs.

• Place 1 tbsp oil in skillet and heat. Add rice slowly, with heat still on, stirring continuously. (This unusual step prevents grains from sticking together.) Pour water into another pot. Bring to boil. Add oil-coated rice slowly and cover pot. Reduce heat to lowest possible setting; set time for 30 minutes. No peeking! (Lifting cover allows steam to escape, and rice won't cook enough.)

Stir-fry mushrooms; set aside. Add rest of oil and stir fry rest of ingredients except for eggs and tamari. After veggies reach prime color, add tamari. Add rice. Stir all. Lightly scramble 2 eggs; add to mixture.

INFECTION

Definition
Invasion and multiplication of unfriendly microorganisms in body tissues.

Causes
The host must be susceptible to the disease, having a compromised immune response, and lacking adequate resistance to the invasion.

    The infectious process is similar to a circular chain with each link representing one of the factors involved in the process. An infectious disease occurs only if each link is present and in proper sequence. Among the links are the causative agent, places where the organism can thrive and reproduce (an open wound, for example), a portal through which the pathogen passes (such as your respiratory system), a mode of transfer, and so on.

Background information
As the great scientists have tried to teach us over the years, *it is not the germ that counts, but the terrain it falls on.*

Medical Validation: The Fiber/Infection Connection
➤*International Journal for Vitamin and Nutrition Research*, 1990. Research was done to determine whether dietary fibers have an immune-defense-stimulating role. The results suggest the possibility that cellulose and pectin may act as such bastions of protection.[131]

➤*Journal of Laboratory and Clinical Medicine*, 1990. The possibility that too much insulin following food consumption plays a role in prolonging convalescence from the flu was explored. Sure enough! Glucose-treated animals had all kinds of problems, from too many free fatty acids to high triglyceride levels. Obviously, these factors delay recuperation.[132]

> Fiber supplementation helps to keep insulin levels stabilized, which in turn helps to prevent secondary problems during any infectious period. This facilitates the healing process.

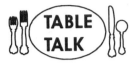

TABLE TALK Don't indulge in fruit juices while recuperating from respiratory diseases. Drink lots of pure water and herbal teas instead. Don't drink regular tea if you're taking aspirin. The tannin content in the tea (a common substance in the bark and fruit of many plants) is an aspirin antagonist, so it's a wipe-out.

➤*American Journal of Tropical Medicine and Hygiene*, 1989. Because this is a particularly significant study, I will include more of the details. Gerbils were maintained on a low-fiber (5%) or a high-fiber (20%) diet in which the major fiber source was cellulose. The animals were inoculated with Giardia lamblia, an intestinal parasite. Animals in the low-fiber diet group were much more likely to become infected than were animals in the high-fiber group. The fiber creates mucus in the gut, entrapping the parasite. Then it travels to the large intestine, where its demise is almost guaranteed.

The fiber content of the diet after inoculation determined the infection rate. When infected animals on the low-fiber diet were placed on the high-fiber diet for twenty-four hours, clearing occurred in the lower small intestine. So, in the case of infections, a high-fiber regimen can be of help even after infection has set in.[133]

Marc Lappé, in his book *Germs That Won't Die*, writes:

Investigators today liken our natural flora to a protective carpet that is an integral part of our anatomy. Remove the carpet, and you strip away one of the critical layers of our body's defense system, leaving us dramatically more vulnerable to infection.

As demonstrated throughout this book, fiber can help to keep that protective "carpet" intact.

IRRITABLE BOWEL AND/OR GASTROINTESTINAL TOLERANCE

Definition
Bowel irregularity—constipation and/or diarrhea, gaseous disten-tion and abdominal pain; a chronic relapsing disorder of aberrant small-bowel motor function.

Causes
Symptoms usually occur in response to various biological and envi-ronmental factors, particularly diets lacking in fiber.

Background information
Irritable bowel syndrome is now treated successfully by merely increasing the fiber content of the diet.[134]

The classic low-residue diet formerly recom-mended for irritable bowel syndrome has been replaced with a high-fiber diet.

Medical Validation: The Fiber/Irritable Bowel Connection
➤*Gastroenterology*, 1990. Dietary fiber supplements modify symp-toms in patients with irritable-bowel syndrome.[135]
➤*Parenteral and Enteral Nutrition*, 1990. Dietary fiber improves gastrointestinal tolerance and bowel function in long-term patients on formula-fed diets, reducing laxative use.[136]
➤*Gastroenterology Clinics of North America*, 1989. Colonic dys-function may be overcome by the gradual addition of combinations of soluble- and insoluble-fiber-containing foods and supplements.[137]
➤*Quarterly Journal of Medicine*, 1989. Treatment with psyllium husk is effective for relieving symptoms and for the maintenance of remission of irritable-bowel syndrome.[138]

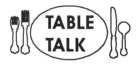

No-Wheat, No-Milk Mini-Marvels
Ingredients: 3 eggs, well beaten; 8 oz. chopped dates or raisins; 1 cup chopped walnuts. • Mix everything together well. Spoon into greased and floured *tiny* muffin tins. Bake at 350°F for 20 minutes. You will have 24 tiny taste treats. *Note*: you *must* use mini-tins.

If one member of the family has digestive disorders, compliance with a high-fiber diet is easier if *everyone* in the family agrees to go on the same diet. The benefits to all will make it more than worth the effort.

➤*Gut*, 1987. Psyllium significantly improves overall well-being in patients with irritable bowel syndrome and in those with constipation. It favorably affects bowel habits and transit time.[139]

➤*Irish Journal of Medical Science*, 1984. A diet composed of 30 grams of fruit and vegetable fiber and 10 grams of cereal fiber was given to patients with irritable bowel syndrome. The result was a significant reduction in abdominal pain and improvement in both bowel habits and state of well-being.[140]

➤*Lancet*, 1977. Fourteen patients placed on 20 grams of bran daily showed a significant reduction in abdominal pain and improvement in bowel habits compared to controls who excluded whole-grain cereal products.[141]

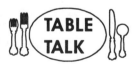

Millet Marvels
Ingredients: 1 cup millet, soaked overnight with water to cover; 1 cup bran; 1 cup flax seed; ½ cup raisins; 1 tbsp cinnamon. • Add other ingredients to millet in the morning. Place in warm oven for 10 minutes.

PROSTATE CANCER

Definition
Cancer of the accessory male reproductive organ. Symptoms of cancer of the prostate are often similar to those of prostate enlargement. If the malignancy is discovered in time, the gland is removed and the cancer doesn't spread.

Causes
Although denied for many years, it is now an accepted fact that diet is a primary cause of cancer.

Background information
One in ten men in this country develops prostate cancer in his lifetime. Twenty thousand prostate cancer cases occur each year in men under the age of 65. Both incidence and mortality of prostate cancer are flourishing.[142]

Prostate cancer is the most common cancer diagnosed in American men and is their second-leading cause of cancer mortality.

Medical Validation: The Fiber/Prostate Cancer Connection
➤*Cancer*, 1989. Increasing consumption of these high-fiber foods—beans, lentils and peas, tomatoes, raisins, dates, and other dried fruit—are all associated with significantly decreased prostate cancer risk among Seventh-Day Adventist men.[143]
➤*International Journal of Epidemiology*, 1988. Population groups with diets high in fiber have a low incidence of cancer, including cancer of the prostate.[144]
➤*Journal of Steroid Biochemistry*, 1987. Fiber intake protects against prostate cancer.[145]
➤*American Journal of Clinical Nutrition*, 1985. Increasing fiber ingestion may modify the risk of prostate cancer.[146]

ULCERS

Definition

A defect or excavation of the surface of an organ or tissue. As commonly used, the term refers to a peptic ulcer of the inner wall, lining of the stomach, or of the duodenum (the first portion of the small intestine).

Causes

While it is known that gastric acid and pepsin are responsible for ulcer formation, precisely why they become troublemakers is not fully understood. Gastric acid is the secretion of glands in the walls of the stomach for use in digestion and pepsin is an enzyme that breaks down protein in food. A new theory relates ulcers to bacteria. Despite all the new knowledge of peptic-ulcer disease, the questions still outnumber the answers. We do know, however, that ulcers can be the product of a poor diet.

Background information

Widespread use of anti-inflammatory drugs has increased the incidence of ulcers, especially in older populations. Serious complications, such as perforation and bleeding, are frequently observed.[147]

> There is a high rate of recurrence after ulcer treatment.

Not long ago, the accepted diet for ulcer patients was a high-fat dairy regimen, intended to coat the stomach with fat to allow healing. As evidenced in the following citations, that view has changed. (*Note*: aloe gel is a workable treatment. The gel, which is aloe juice thickened by Irish moss, slows transit, allowing the aloe to coat the gastrointestinal tract and heal the ulcer.)

This is a life-threatening disease, yet peptic ulcers remain silent in a substantial number of patients, refusing to announce their presence with symptoms until a very advanced state.

Medical Validation: The Fiber/Ulcer Connection

➤*Gut*, 1990. There is an association between duodenal ulceration and low-fiber intake.[148]

➤*Revista Espanola de las Enfermedades del Aparato Digestivo*, 1989. The ulcer index is found to be smaller in those treated with rice oil (derived from rice bran) than in controls.[149]

➤*Clinical Science*, 1987. Fresh rice bran can significantly reduce ulcers. Similarly, unmilled rice is protective by significantly reducing the ulcer incidence.[150]

➤*Surgery, Gynecology and Obstetrics*, 1987. During a thirty-hour treatment period, test animals fed guar gum showed a lower number of ulcers than controls fed normal food. Guar gum increases the healing rate. The mechanisms suggested for ulcer prevention and increased ulcer healing rate may be due to reduced acidity, increased local mucosal supply of energy, and mechanical protection as a result of guar-gum feeding.[151]

➤*Lancet*, 1982. Seventy-three people with recently healed duodenal ulcers changed their diets. About half ate a great deal of whole-grain bread and whole cereals, plus lots of vegetables. The others were asked to avoid these foods. Those who ate the least amount of fiber developed new ulcers within six months.[152]

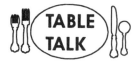

The Ulcer-Fighting Soup
Ingredients: 2 quarts water; ½ cup rice or barley; ½ cup each: diced onion, green pepper, celery, carrot, sweet potato, zucchini, mushrooms; 2 tbsp tamari; dash pepper; clove garlic; oregano; thyme. • Bring water to boil. Add rice (or barley). Reduce heat and cover. Cook on low for ½ hour. Add tamari and vegetables and seasonings. Barely simmer for 1 to 2 hours, or until you are ready to eat. Remove garlic clove before serving.

VARICOSE VEINS

Definition

Swollen veins. Veins susceptible to swelling and distortion lie under the skin near the surface of the legs.

Causes

This condition is due to the malfunction of valves that normally ensure the flow of blood through veins and back up to the heart. Burkitt likens the mechanism to a pump forcing water uphill. The pump pushes the water up and the valves prevent its return. Straining to pass small firm stools is a major cause, forcing blood back down the leg veins, allowing the valves to become defective.

Background information

Sixty-four percent of women over fifty have varicose veins. That's a lot of women running around with veins they don't want on display. Needless to say, it doesn't just happen on your fiftieth birthday. The process starts decades earlier. Burkitt explains:

> *Varicose veins are rare among people under the age of twenty but become progressively more common with increasing age. This suggests that the cause lies in a progressive and cumulative effect of some environmental factor operating over a long period of time. Animals do not suffer from varicose veins, which indicates that the basic cause must be something in the way of life peculiar to human beings. The evidence thus suggests that inadequate fiber in our diet is an important cause of varicose veins.*

Medical Validation: The Fiber/Varicose Vein Connection

➢*Journal of the Royal Society of Health*, 1985. There were fewer cases of varicose veins among seventy-five lifelong vegetarians than control groups studied.[153]

As with hiatus hernia, review the validation cited under CONSTIPATION.

MISCELLANEOUS PROBLEMS

A few other medical disturbances and their links with fiber deserve attention.

Acne and other skin conditions

The Western diet is associated with an increased incidence of acne, as cited in several observational studies. Far less acne is found among the black population in Zambia eating traditional diets than among young blacks in the United States.[154] In an experimental study, patients show rapid clearing of acne following supplementation with one ounce daily of a bran cereal.[155]

Treatment of any skin condition is always more effective when the intestinal tract is free of disease-producing fungi. Vegetable fiber is recommended to reduce yeast colonies between your intestinal villi—the threadlike projections covering the surface of the mucous membranes lining your small intestine which serve as the absorption sites of nutrients. Fiber also helps to avoid yeast cells from invading your lymph tract and circulating blood. This is effective in clearing seborrheic eczema (the kind that causes excessive discharge from the sebaceous glands, forming greasy scales or cheesy plugs) and other skin conditions.[156]

Crohn's disease

Dietary fiber has proved effective in decreasing symptoms of Crohn's disease in a few clinical studies.[157] Crohn's disease is a dangerous intestinal inflammation of the ileum (the lower portion of the small intestine).

Food intolerance

The efficacy of increasing food tolerance with the addition of guar gum is clearly demonstrated.[158] Meal supplementation with guar gum improves glucose tolerance.[159]

Menstruation problems

One study evaluates nutrient intake in several non-athletic college women with light periods, compared with women who have the more usual menstrual problems. The groups did not differ in any aspect of body composition, body weight, age of menarche (start of menstruation), or perceived psychological stress. Among other factors, *the women with light periods, free of pain, are found to consume significantly more fiber!*[160]

Some women who adopt high-fiber diets are at less risk for breast cancer, but appear to be at greater risk for menstrual-cycle dysfunction *if* their diets do not encourage normal circulating estrogen concentrations! High-fiber, low-fat diets are the answer, not high-fiber, *no-fat* diets. Fat, as found in intact foods, is an important nutrient. Our brains are comprised of more fat than protein. Fats govern most of the vital functions of humans. It's not difficult to learn the difference between *fat, the nutrient* (as found in whole foods) and *fat, the precursor of disease* (as found in processed foods).

Ovarian cancer

The effect of a high-fiber diet on estrogen levels was investigated in healthy premenopausal women. Levels of a steroid hormone (estrone sulphate) were lower when compared with women on typical Western diets.[161]

Pancreatic cancer

A study reported in 1990 in the *International Journal of Cancer* noted a reduced risk of pancreatic cancer associated with consumption of fiber from fruit, vegetable, and cereal sources.[162]

Triglycerides

Triglycerides are storage fatty acids, which, when in excess, are considered as dangerous as high cholesterol levels. Unlike most of the medical conditions discussed so far, elevated triglyceride levels appear to be more resistant to change with dietary fiber. It does happen, however, in certain circumstances.

Feeding test animals a diet rich in fermentable carbohydrate (the kind of fiber that breaks down in the cecum, described in Chapter 2), decreases triglycerides as well as cholesterol, even when the animals are fed lard and other cholesterol-raising substances.[163] Fiber may offer protection against an increase in triglyceride levels in those who are consuming large amounts of sugar.[164]

SUMMARY

Persuasive arguments are no longer necessary to convince anyone of the influence of dietary fiber and health, but only because of hard-won knowledge. Information about the beneficial effects of fiber came later than was necessary to objective scientists. They could have learned from the practitioners who have been using these concepts over the years, or they could have asked great-grandma. She has always known that "roughage" unlocks wellness. The wisdom of the ages!

Whatever else nature may lack, it doesn't lack experience. We can no longer define malnourishment as food shortage. You can easily be simultaneously overfed and undernourished on low-fiber, overprocessed American convenience food. You can also easily nurture yourself back to health.

EXTRA!!! The Times EXTRA!!!

Degenerative disease is avoidable. It is also curable. Treatment is dietary/lifestyle.

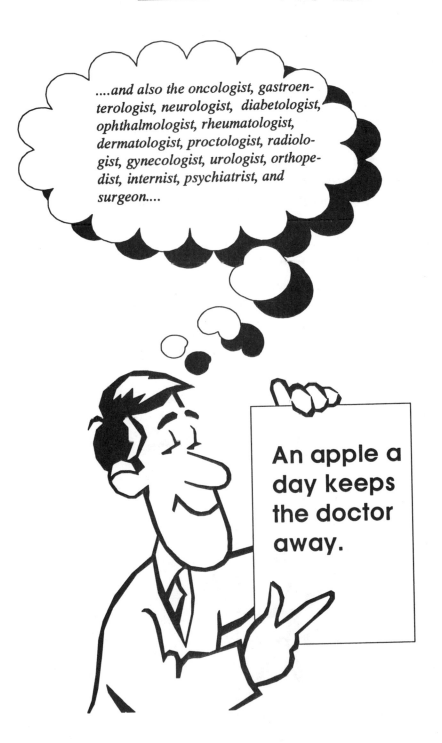

Eating is one of the pleasures of life. This is a concept which should never be forgotten. People generally will not eat a nutritious food unless it is in a pleasing and acceptable form. With a little effort at first, you can learn to prepare meals that are both delicious and nutritious.

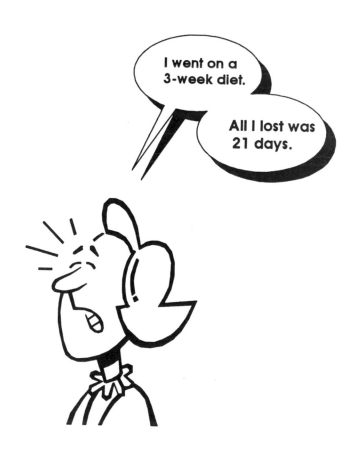

CHAPTER 4

FIBER
HOW IT AFFECTS WEIGHT

Stories in novels are usually so different from life as I know it, just as the promises in diet books turn out to be little more than imagination. The diet-book messages, however, would be less fantasy and more reality if we could, (1) change human nature and, (2) alter the biological pathways we've inherited down through the ages.

But we're a pleasure-bent society *and* we're stuck with particular metabolic pathways. We are designed for survival in a different social format with different dietary parameters—effective for an era when it was possible to miss food for long periods of time, an era that was pre-agricultural, pre-farming. The genetic imprint of yesteryear is a major roadblock in coping with influences which present-day lifestyles exert on body weight. You can, however, work *with*, not *against*, your Paleolithic heritage. Getting back to ancient foodways can be as simple as adding more fiber to your diet.

THE BAD NEWS

Because we are not always rational animals, yet remain incurably biological, the past several decades have seen a steadily increasing proportion of overweight adults in the United States, especially among women.[1] Here are some of the reasons why:

Food alterations. Diet patterns have changed and continue to change; the distance between a natural food and food on the table is widening.

Fat cell metabolism. Fat cells are economical and efficient in energy storage. We have the ability to stockpile fat easily—to maintain important metabolic processes during famine and to help provide energy for hunting the saber-toothed tiger.

Present pleasures. It's hard to give up a present pleasure for a future benefit. We are programmed to respond to instant gratification without consideration of future problems.

Emotional responses. The "sweet reward" is universal; it is part of every culture, and is offered as a bonus for special behavior, or as a stress-reliever—but not necessarily to satisfy hunger.

Low blood sugar and your hypothalamus appestat. Low blood sugar causes your stomach to increase the speed and force of its contractions. It also increases the sensitivity of your taste buds. And it motivates your hypothalamus to send impulses which step up production of gastric juices and saliva. Even more significant, low blood sugar activates a particular portion of your hypothalamus called the *satiety center*, or *appestat*.

The hypothalamus (Greek for *under the inner room*) lies near the underside of your brain, just about in the center of your head. Not much bigger than a small prune, this incredible mass of cells acts as the command post of your brain. The appestat controls your appetite by communicating with your brain.[2] When this hunger indicator is activated by falling blood sugar, and perhaps by a mild sensation of fatigue, it sets a chain of events in motion. The final demand is: FEED ME! NOW!

Feedback systems promote efficient fat storage and signal your brain to seek food when your body *thinks* it is needed, not necessarily when it is actually needed.

Physiological responses. A five-month-old human fetus will increase its swallowing rate when a sweetener is injected into the amniotic fluid of the mother.[3] This suggests that humans prefer sweets long before birth. Theories, and only theories, abound as to why we desire and respond to a sweet stimulus.

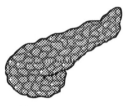

Pancreas

An unpleasant taste stimulus (like broccoli for George Bush) has a significantly different effect on the character and volume of pancreatic flow than a pleasant stimulus (like broccoli for me!).[4] Pleasant taste stimuli affect the activity and the secretions along the digestive tract.

Serotonin deficiency. When a behavior-regulating neurotransmitter called *serotonin* is out of order, it causes you to binge, uncurbed. (Neurotransmitters are vehicles for communication between your nerve cells.) The result is excessive consumption of refined carbohydrates, and/or cravings for sweets.[5,6] Carbohydrate cravings can represent a deficiency of serotonin, rather than an actual need for food.[7] (So here's your biological and scientific excuse for excessive consumption of ice cream—or maybe it's chocolate. For me it's pecan pie; sometimes cheese cake.)

Many people who have allergies have difficulty controlling weight. The problem is one of biochemical internal disarray caused by the food allergy, which interferes with the natural "set point." The complex brain tries to sort this out, along with other confusing, outdated messages.

Seduction in the supermarket. A group of rats was given a choice of their usual fare or American supermarket snack foods. The animals chose biscuits, chocolates, and marshmallows in preference to regular chow (exhibiting rather human characteristics). In 60 days, they gained 78 grams of weight, which, for a rat, is a lot.[8] Yes, even a rat can be seduced in the supermarket.

We are bombarded with attractive advertisements for foods which are devoid of fiber. The more a food is processed, the more profitable it is for the manufacturer. Compare the cost of a potato with that of potato chips, weight for weight. It is no surprise that if a pound of good-quality baking potatoes costs about 59 cents, you will pay almost four dollars for a pound of potato chips. Deficiencies or excesses of nutrients cause your cells to ask in their wordless language, *what happened*? And then they answer the only way they know how, the way they've been responding across the centuries by using techniques meant for a time that predates food processing and the availability of 4,000 foods in your supermarket, usually located not more than a few blocks or short drive away.

Why Apple Juice Causes Weight Gain

High technology has recently helped to uncover a huge mass of new information. We are beginning to learn exactly when, why, and how fat gets deposited in adipose (fat) tissue. Enzyme activity can now be examined within fat cells and changes have been recorded as they take place in those who are overweight and also during weight loss. This knowledge, previously unknown, is very useful.

We now know that one enzyme in fat tissue sends a message to your brain to increase caloric intake as soon as weight loss takes place. Thanks a lot! Most of us could do without the zeal of this interfering enzyme which regulates our "fat" affairs. Such control creates a catch-22 situation, perhaps explaining why we struggle during weight loss, sustaining a persistent message of hunger.

Here's the important part: TOO MUCH INSULIN INITIATES COMMUNICATION BETWEEN THIS ENZYME AND YOUR BRAIN.[9] Every surge of glucose absorbed brings a corresponding surge of inslin release. Insulin is the key to getting glucose into your cells. Glucose supplies your cells with fuel to do its work, to keep you alive, to give you energy. It's your fuel for both immediate and future needs. Without glucose, your body won't move. But when glucose is absorbed beyond a certain rate, the ability of your liver to store the glucose (as glycogen) for future use is exceeded, *and the surplus is converted to fat.*

You can see how insulin metabolism affects weight control. Any dietary change that leads to more rapid absorption of carbohydrate and greater insulin release is likely to promote obesity. Removing fiber from a natural high-carbohydrate food dumps too much sugar into your blood, causing the production of too much insulin.[10] *Fiber doesn't exist in apple juice.*

> Refined carbohydrates are responsible for much of our obesity. Is it the high percentage of sugar or the lack of fiber? As the song goes, *you can't have one without the other.*

More About Fiber-Free Foods And Weight

It has long since been suggested that refined carbohydrates are responsible for most of the obesity in technological societies.[11] In 1956, this hypothesis was demonstrated scientifically. Test animals were fed "purified" corn starch. These animals had fat deposits weighing twice as much as those fed whole corn.[12] Processed foods are easier to eat. Additional experiments reveal that foods requiring little effort to consume are swallowed more readily and in greater quantities. Again, refined carbohydrates translate to lack of fiber.

Feed healthy adults equal amounts of fat in the form of whole peanuts, peanut butter and peanut oil, and more fat is absorbed from the peanut oil than from the peanut butter, and more from the peanut butter than from the peanuts. Why? Fiber blocks the absorption of fat—and hence calories—in the intestines. The more the product is refined, the more fiber is removed, and the less "fat-blocking" occurs.

If it takes 17.2 minutes to eat a quantity of whole apples, it will take only 1.5 minutes to consume an equicaloric amount of apple juice.[13] The consumption of a large meal of whole wheat bread takes 45 minutes, as compared with 34 minutes for an equicaloric amount of white bread. When participants are asked to eat bread until they feel comfortably full, ten out of twelve eat less whole-grain bread.[14]

Needless to say, when a solid food is converted to liquid, the difference in the rate of consumption is even greater. This is true whether the meal is drunk or pumped into your mouth.[15] When you drink a beverage sweetened with sugar, you don't have to work at all to get your carbohydrate load. And you consume more of a beverage through straws with larger holes than through straws with smaller openings.[16] Similarly, you eat more shelled nuts than unshelled.[17]

> WE INGEST MORE FOOD WHEN ITS FIBER IS REMOVED.

Exercise Is Not Always The Answer

Well, let's modify that heading. We've been told again and again: if you really want to lose weight and keep it off, you've got *to get off your tail and exercise.*

Exercise is a significant answer when we exercise up to our excess calorie intake. Judging

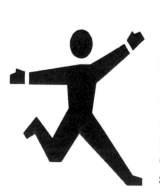 from our overweight status, that's not happening. Few of us burn up all the calories we ingest, and the excess gets stored as fat.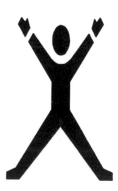

Why should exercise play such a dominant role in weight loss? Is lack of exercise the *cause* of our obesity epidemic in the first place? The fact that we are a less-mobile society is significant. Weight gain is due to many complex factors which are difficult to generalize for an entire population.

We are not always overweight because of lack of exercise. Of course exercise is a factor; exercise is beneficial; exercise helps you to absorb nutrients more efficiently; and, yes, you will lose weight if you exercise to the degree that you "use up" more than you "take in." But the amount of movement to accomplish that goal is hard to come by, and exercise is not the only ingredient. (Don't you know at least a few people who are physically active, yet overweight, and at least one person who is skinny, yet inactive?)

Very often women in particular reduce their food intake after initiating an exercise program. This results in a decrease in the quality of nutrient consumption from their diets, adding to difficulties.[18]

And that's all the bad news.

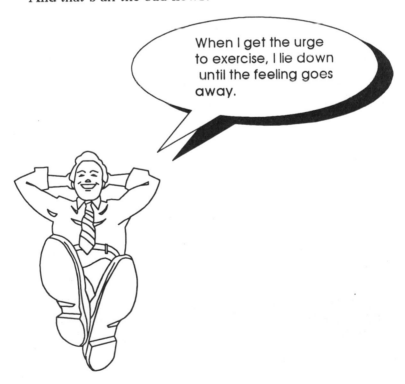

When I get the urge to exercise, I lie down until the feeling goes away.

THE GOOD NEWS

Here's the good news: The greater your fiber consumption, the higher your caloric waste. Fiber causes a true alteration in digestion and absorption of fat. Part of the fat becomes "associated" with fiber so that it is unavailable for digestion and increases fat excretion.[19]

Even better news is that you can manage a high-fiber intake without making major adjustments to your usual eating regimen. But that's Chapter 5. This discussion is about *how* fiber interacts with calories and your weight.

Fiber And Satiety

When you consume enough fiber, both your small and large intestines contain more watery material. When your bowels are full, you do not feel empty. You stop eating when a certain degree of satiety is achieved. Different foods offer varying levels of satiety.

The apple experiment demonstrates that food is less satisfying when it is depleted of fiber. Here are the details of the satiety part of that experiment:

Volunteers were presented with test meals of 482 grams of raw apples, eaten whole except for cores and stalks, and of 469 grams of juice made from the same batch of apples. The nutrient content of the two meals was the same. Immediately after the meal, the average satiety score was determined. Significantly higher "feel-full" totals were reported after eating apples than after drinking juice, and the difference continued for two hours.

Subsequently, the researchers compared meals of oranges and orange juice of equal caloric content, and also of grapes and grape juice. Again, the fruits evoked consistently higher satiety scores than did the juice.[20]

Does chewing explain the satisfying effect of the whole apple? Since purée of apples evokes a higher satiety score than apple juice, chewing is not the entire explanation for the satisfying effect of fiber. The water-holding properties of fiber make your gut contents bulkier, and this distension of your stomach and small intestine induces satiety. Another possibility is that fiber changes the pattern of your hormone release, thereby preventing low blood sugar, which contributes to hunger signals, as explained above.[21,22]

> Slowed transit through your mouth and stomach (the area of your body where *unhurried* transit is good) may delay nutrient absorption and produce a sensation of satiety.

LEVEL OF SATIETY ON A 0-10 SCALE AFTER MEALS OF FRUIT AND FRUIT JUICES

	Apples	Oranges	Grapes
Fruit ≻	6.9	6.4	4.2
Juice ≻	1.4	1.5	0.8

Adapted from Table 1, in Heaton W. "Food intake regulation and fiber," in *Medical Aspects of Dietary Fiber*, GA Spiller, and RM Kay, (Eds). New York, Plenum Medical Book Co, 1980, p 227.

The juice used in the study reported in the chart above was made from the same batch of fruit in each case. The fruit and juice meals were chemically the same except for the absence of fiber in the juices. Note that the higher the natural sugar content in the original fruit, the less the level of satiety—even with consumption of intact food.

In unprocessed plant foods, carbohydrates are always embedded in fiber. (Honey may be the one exception.) Fiber supplementation is an attempt to return the carbohydrates in your diet to a more natural state.

As Burkitt explains, the type of obesity common to Western cultures occurs when someone slowly develops an extra fourteen pounds of fat over fifteen years, from twenty-five to forty years of age. This is one pound per year, which can occur if only about 40 extra calories out of the intake of about 2000 are stored each day, representing only 2 per cent extra compared with requirements. Fiber is the only constituent in our daily diet that contains no calories. If a high-fiber diet decreases energy absorbed from 1 to 2 percent, it seems reasonable to assume that fiber-rich food will help to keep a person slim.

Validation: Studies On Fiber Intake And Weight Loss

➤*International Journal of Obesity*, 1990. Dietary fiber has proved beyond all doubt to be of value in the management of overweight, in helping weight loss, and in shrinking hunger feelings.[23]

➤*International Journal of Obesity*, 1990. Dietary fiber added to a very low-calorie diet helps by reducing hunger and increasing the number of eliminations. This has no effect on nutrient absorption.[24]

➤*Journal of Nutrition*, 1990. Consumption of soluble fiber results in smaller final body weight. The effect is related to the insulin response of the dietary component.[25]

➤*International Journal of Obesity*, 1990. A supplement of dietary fiber added to a very low-calorie diet reduces hunger and increases the number of bowel movements, without impairment of nutrient absorption.[26]

➤*Ugeskrift for Laeger*, 1990. Using a fiber food with a very low-calorie diet improves compliance with the diet by normalizing hunger and increasing the incidence of elimination without diminishing the metabolism of nutrients.[27]

➤*American Journal of Clinical Nutrition*, 1989. Cereals containing relatively large quantities of dietary fiber may decrease short-term food intake.[28]

➤*Journal of Nutrition*, 1989. Meals containing various doses of guar gum were ingested by healthy subjects after a twelve-hour fast. After eating, the rise in blood glucose was higher without the guar than with it. Increased doses led to a smaller rise in insulin. Guar gum is found to reduce the variation in glucose responses between individuals, as well as the initial rate of gastric emptying.

> The glycemic advantage of guar gum is lost after the heating and homogenization necessary for canning.[29]

➤*Magnesium Research*, 1989. In obese test animals, a high-fiber diet reduces body weight and also returns magnesium levels to normal.[30]

➤*Geriatrics*, 1989. The most important dietary precept for elderly patients with diabetes is the maintenance of desirable body weight. It is now proposed that the diet prescribed contains those carbohydrates that are primarily complex and rich in fiber. This study concludes with a critical message: *"The nutritional program outlined is a good program for everyone, and the entire family is encouraged to participate in the meal planning and preparation involved."*[31]

> Dietary guidelines for diabetic patients are not fundamentally different from those for any other person desiring weight loss and a healthful diet.

➤*Appetite*, 1986. Overweight people consume only a little more than half the fiber recommended, contributing to failure of weight loss— despite having received instruction on the rationale of a high-fiber diet. Difficulties in compliance are common.[32]

➤*British Journal of Nutrition*, 1984: Soluble fiber reduces hunger and influences carbohydrate and lipid (fat) metabolism in a beneficial way.[33]

➤*Dietary Fiber in Health and Disease*, 1982. Obese patients with diabetes do not complain of hunger on high-fiber diets which provide as little as 800 calories a day.[34]

➤*Medical Aspects of Dietary Fiber*, 1980. The greater your fiber consumption, the higher your waste of calories. Energy output is increased with the bulking action of dietary fiber. The precise source of this energy is vague, but it represents a further way in which fiber prevents energy intake from exceeding output.[35]

SUMMARY

The message is loud and clear: The best way to slow your eating pace is to consume fiber-rich foods (especially raw foods). Does this mean we must turn eating habits back 50 or 100 years? We all know such dietary change in today's world is easier said than done. It's difficult to eat old-fashioned foods in our high-tech, fast-lane world.

While we try to learn new ways to shop and to cook and fashionable ways to be selective in restaurants, be aware that in the late twentieth century, *fiber is available in supplemental form, offered to enhance health and/or as a feel-full helper.* High-quality fiber supplements utilize more than one type of fiber. Remember that fiber is a complex substance that stimulates different types of intestinal activity, depending on the source. Who can say what form of fiber is best? But we do know that a varied quality-fiber potpourri offers greater health and weight-loss advantages.

Concentrated fiber preparations are effective for weight loss *provided the doses consumed are large enough.*[36] The availability of fiber supplements reflect transitions that have come about because we are learning how to link nutrition and health. One thing is certain: The higher the percentage of fiber in your diet, the lower the tape-measure reading around your waist.

CALORIES PER GRAM OF DIETARY FIBER: POPULAR READY-TO-EAT CEREALS & NUTS

100-GRAM BASIS (ABOUT 3½ OUNCES)

Food Item	Dietary Fiber (grams)	Calories Per Gram Dietary Fiber
All-Bran	29.90	8.33
Figs	16.99	15.95
Dates	8.75	30.97
Shredded wheat	9.30	37.85
Wheaties	7.00	49.86
Grape Nuts Flakes	6.40	55.94
Nutri-Grain, Barley	5.80	64.14
Cheerios	3.80	102.89
Almonds	5.30	112.83
Walnuts (English)	5.20	125.38
Corn Chex	1.80	217.78
Product 19	1.10	346.36
Corn Flakes	1.10	353.64
Apple Jacks	.90	430.00
Special K	.80	487.50
Froot Loops	.80	490.00
Frosted Rice Krispies	.20	1915.00
Rice Crispies	.20	1975.00

Source: California Dried Fig Advisory Board, Fresno, California

The relationship between the stimulation of insulin and weight gain has been confirmed time and again. Appetite or subjective feelings of hunger are connected with low blood glucose levels. Since fiber helps to "quiet" insulin reactions, which in turn stabilizes glucose levels, consuming fiber is a metabolic advantage in terms of weight stability.

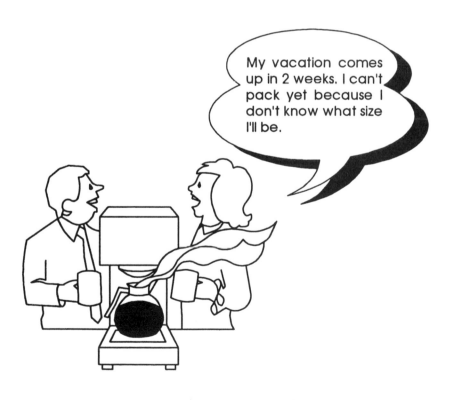

My vacation comes up in 2 weeks. I can't pack yet because I don't know what size I'll be.

CHAPTER 5

FIBER
HOW TO GET IT

"Eat your vegetables!" Who would have thought we would hear this command stated even more emphatically in our adult years than when we were kids? A survey cited in the *American Journal of Public Health* noted that 22 percent of Americans consume no vegetables; 45 percent do not eat any fruit.[1] Worse, only 9 percent have servings of both fruit and vegetables as recommended by the United States Department of Agriculture and Department of Health and Human Services. An additional concern is that the choice of vegetables among this small percentage lacks *variety*.

If all that isn't bad enough, diets which do include at least three servings of vegetables and two servings of fruit contain only about 17 grams of dietary fiber—less than half of what many experts suggest as minimally desirable.

Additional research is just as discouraging. Where two thousand well-educated individuals were questioned, more than 90 percent were unaware of the recommendations for consuming fiber. Nor did they know which cereals were high in fiber, or just how far up "high" should be.[2] Other studies support the fact that the ability to apply fiber know-how does not match the level of nutrition knowledge. *Fiber literacy rarely correlates with fiber consumption.*[3] Yet another study shows that fiber compliance is lower than vitamin compliance.[4]

Most government health agencies are advocating a doubling or tripling of fiber intake. Typical recommendations are set at 30 to 50 grams of dietary fiber daily.[5] Fiber facts must be put into perspective and practice. Now that you know how important fiber is for your health, let's examine options for increasing fiber intake.

FIBER FROM FOOD

Here's a high-fiber regimen followed by a group of monks living a stress-free life in a beautiful mountain retreat in Oregon:

Breakfast: Buckwheat porridge with sesame seed milk, mixed berries, an assortment of rehydrated dried fruit. Fresh fruit; sprouted lentils; flax seed.

Lunch: Raw foods: tomatoes, cucumbers, minced carrots, green and red peppers, green leafy vegetables, cabbage; fermented mixed vegetables; mixed salads of: steamed or raw beets, potatoes, parsley, sprouted fenugreek seeds, garlic; cultured-milk product.

Dinner: Raw foods, mixed salads and a hot soup boiled from roots and vegetables. Soup is served with bread (buckwheat rolls, crisp hard rye bread, or Essene—which is sprouted wheat or rye bread).

Snacks: Fruit, nuts and seeds, sprouted legumes.

Isn't it too bad that the majority of us can't maintain this kind of dietary pattern if we chose to? MOST OF US ARE TOO ACCUS-TOMED TO THE INSTANT BIRTH OF A MEAL AND TO SHELF-LIFE FOODS TO BE ABLE TO MAKE THIS MENU WORK IN THE REAL WORLD! It is my hope that you will at least try to be more selective where and when possible and that you will attempt some of the recipes outlined in previous chapters. For reasons cited later in this chapter, another measure should be the addition of fiber supplementation.

Look at the fiber content of foods with which you are more familiar. When checking food-fiber values, be sure to use newer reference guides which consider *total* dietary fiber. Older food tables do not include the soluble fibers. Some of the fiber values of common foods are listed in Appendix C.

Don't be taken in by advertising hype. Eating bran muffins won't do the job. *Nine* bran muffins a day have no effect on lipid levels in either normal people or those with high cholesterol.[6] Thomas' oat-bran muffins contain a mere 2.9 grams of fiber, and Hostess oat-bran muffins even less. And who needs all the calories, processed fat, and sweetening agents that go along for the bran-muffin ride?

You can cook *real* oatmeal for 7.7 grams of fiber per bowl, buckwheat (kasha) for 9.6 grams, or brown rice for 5.5. You can also learn a few tricks to expedite preparations.

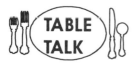 Place cereal grains in a thermos of hot water at night. Your bowl of cereal will be ready and waiting for breakfast.

Compare the fiber values of whole grains with Instant Quaker Oats, which has 2 grams. Note that there is far more sugar than oat bran in Post Honey Bunches of Oats. You'd have to eat 28 servings to end up with as much oat bran as you'd get in one bowl of hot oat-bran cereal.

With a little planning, you can go the whole-foods route without upsetting your time schedule. Examples:

~ When I travel, I order oatmeal and sliced banana in restaurants for breakfast; no hot milk or sugared cinnamon, thank you.

~ It only takes a minute or two to change the water in the pot of kidney beans you soaked overnight (10 grams), in preparation for dinner. When you get home from work, you can cook the beans slowly over a low temperature. If this appears to be a lot of time and work, prepare this meal in triplicate over the weekend and freeze.

~ Maybe you could scrub potatoes ahead (4 1/2 grams per long potato), so they're ready for baking at 6:00 PM. (Do you eat while watching *Wheel of Fortune*?) Wash and cut the veggies for steaming, too. A long carrot yields 2.3 grams of fiber; broccoli spears about 3 grams for a good-sized portion; asparagus 1.7 for a half cup; 2.5 for a half cup of beets. Pick your favorites. I know of no shortcuts for an ongoing supply of fresh vegetables, but I think it's worth the effort.

~ You can assemble a big salad, and plan on fruit for dessert. Leaf veggies consist mostly of water, so you'd better prepare a lot! Unless you are willing to put together a kitchen-sink salad, you won't get too much fiber from this part of your meal. But, although they are not heavy-weights as fiber sources, salad vegetables offer good nutrition.

> An entire head of lettuce contains only 1.6 grams of fiber.

Even if you follow these food suggestions (and I hope you do), your total fiber intake will still fall short of optimal. That's why I also recommend fiber supplementation. High-fiber diets meeting the 50-gram quota may be too austere for all but the most highly motivated. It's obvious that such an approach cannot work for everyone in today's fast-forward world. But knowledge is the beginning of change.

Food and Fiber Facts

Don't be discouraged if you can't go "all out" and even *approach* the monk's diet. You can still be selective when making food choices. Health is not a black-or-white condition. Be choosy at the supermarket, in the restaurant, at the business conference, when visiting friends. Do the best you can with what's easy and available. Keep the concept in mind; *get as much fiber with the least amount of calories.*

In addition to *Table Talk* suggestions scattered throughout the chapters, here are a few more facts that may be helpful.

➤Crunchy foods are not always fiber-rich. Lettuce and celery are low-fiber sources; so is cabbage. Peas have lots of fiber; so does broccoli.

➤The calorie value of a potato is slightly more than an apple and slightly less than a pear, but offers a generous amount of fiber. It's the butter, the oils, and the sauces that make potatoes fattening.

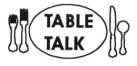 When you prepare dinner, throw a sweet potato or two into the oven. Let them sit around after they're cooked, and hold them in abeyance until you are looking for a tasty, filling, and tempting snack later on in the evening. This more than satisfies any sweet tooth.

➤A whole sugar beet provides only one teaspoonful of refined sugar, so sugar, of course, has no fiber. It isn't easy to avoid the use of refined sugar. Grate regular beets and other root veggies into your salads.

➤When looking to satisfy your sweet tooth, nibble on prunes, dates, and especially figs. When prunes replace grape juice—each having the same amount of simple sugars—the prunes increase your fiber intake; the grape juice won't. Prunes reduce bile-acid concentration; grape juice doesn't.[7]

---

2 dates contain 1.2 grams of fiber
3 prunes contain 1.9 grams of fiber
1 fig contains 2 grams of fiber

➤Rye bread contains white flour with a few grains of rye thrown in, not for good measure, but for good sales. A cup of white flour contains 1.6 grams of fiber. Compare that to the fiber content before wheat is processed, which is 14.4 grams per cup—the same quantity of fiber in one cup of whole rye.

➤"Wheat" or even "whole wheat" on a label does not necessarily mean that the flour is all, or even significantly, whole grain. (Nabisco Whole Wheat Premium Plus Saltines, Nabisco Wheatsworth, and Pepperidg Farm Hearty Wheat crackers all contain more white flour than whole-wheat flour.)

➤The term "unbleached flour" has nothing to do with fiber content. Stone-grinding, however, does not remove fiber, minerals, or vitamins. When purchasing grain products (bread, crackers, etc.) look for the stone-ground label. A slice of Pepperidge Farm Multi-Grain bread contains only 1 gram of fiber, the same amount as found in Arnold Country White. Don't be misled by fancy titles.

➤Fiber in most foods will be reduced by long-term cooking and by the high-heat process used in canning.[8] Some foods, however, must be cooked in order to burst the cell walls to free any nutrients. Potatoes are one example.

> 1 cup of hot Wheatena cereal contains 3.6 grams of fiber; 1 cup of Wheaties has 2 grams

➤Another major consideration is calories. Heartland cereal offers 4.7 grams of fiber in a portion, but has 92 calories per gram of fiber! Corn flakes? About 2 grams in a serving, with 185 calories per gram of fiber. All-Bran is a better choice, at 30 grams of fiber per portion with only 8.33 calories per gram. Beware Frosted Rice Krinkles, at a tenth of a gram of fiber per portion, translating to a whopping 3850 calories per gram of fiber! (See Chart on page 101 for more comparisons.)

➤Although nuts are high in fiber, they are often available only in a detrimental form: salted, overprocessed, and rancid. The higher the oil content, the more quickly a food gets rancid. Nuts, of course, are very high in oil. Once shelled, the rancidity process accelerates rapidly. For this reason, nuts should be purchased in the shell.

> Almonds are among the most stable of nuts and are not as offending as most other nuts after shelling.

➤Sprouts are the least contaminated, treated, and processed food available to you. Much scientific evidence indicates that sprouting a seed or bean enhances its already high nutritional value. Sprouting increases the nutrient content of some seeds and beans by up to 600 percent or more. It's easy to sprout lentils, chickpeas, adzuki beans, and green peas. These high-fiber sources can be growing in your kitchen right up to the moment you prepare your meal. (Sprouts should be a major component of a kitchen-sink salad.)

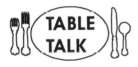 Sprouted-grain breads, known as *Essene* or *Manna* breads, are especially good. Try the ones with cinnamon and/or fruits and nuts, or seeds. For those who are wheat-sensitive, *not to worry*. The sprouting process changes a food, and many people who cannot tolerate regular wheat products rarely have difficulty with sprouted-grain breads—provided all the grains in the bread are sprouted.

➤Yogurt does not have a full range of nutrients and has absolutely no fiber. It should never be consumed alone. Combining yogurt with raspberries (when in season) fills the missing links. Try pears or bananas when raspberries are not available. Because yogurt is a fermented product, its nutrient value is increased. Fermentation adds healthful bacteria.

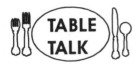 **Seed Balls**
Ingredients: 2 green peppers; 1 bunch celery; 3 shredded zucchini; 1 bunch green onions; 1 yellow onion; 1 bunch parsley; 1 cup ground sunflower seeds; 1 cup ground sesame seeds; 1 tbsp basil; 1 tbsp caraway seed. • Mince veggies finely . Add seeds and spices; blend well. Form into balls. Place on warming tray for 6 hours or in oven at lowest setting for 4 hours.

FIBER FROM SUPPLEMENTS

Fiber supplements can contain naturally-occurring plant fiber or synthetic fiber.[9] The synthetic fibers possess little of the fermentive and biological properties of plant fibers which normally occur in the human diet.[10]

The kind of extradietary fibers used in health-food supplements are the naturally-occurring plant fibers. I refer to this kind of supplementation as *fiber-food.* The formulas are derived from plants which are basically old-fashioned foods, but are cloaked in late twentieth-century technology. Such a formula can enhance your well-being, and, in addition to convenience, offer certain advantages. Here are a baker's dozen benefits.

(1) The presence of a plant cell wall matrix (that is, the fiber) in a food can provide a physical barrier to digestion. Most of the pectin and hemicellulose is within that plant cell wall and is difficult for enzymes to reach. So an intact cell wall may slow the penetration of digestive enzymes.[11] Consequently, grinding of the fiber source to very fine particle size may disrupt the cell wall structure sufficiently to make digestible nutrients more available.[12] Powdered or blended fibers have this advantage.

(2) The *American Journal of Clinical Nutrition* advises that "Cooked bran has no significant effect on intestinal transit time. The cereal manufacturing process alters wheat bran so that when cooked, it has less effect on the intestine than does a comparable amount of raw bran. Fiber supplements that increase transit speed may have different implications even though they share the common property of bulk expanders."[13]

(3) Fruit may be off-limits for anyone with blood sugar problems (hypoglycemia or diabetes). Foods that are too high in sugar, even natural sugar, can be deleterious for many people, in spite of fiber content. Pectin, the valuable fiber in fruit, has proved to be health-effective in isolated form. The goodies in your fruit bowl contain varying amounts of pectin, depending on ripeness and growing conditions. A high-quality fiber supplement offers standardized availability of pectin.

(4) Fibers vary in function. Many cause beneficial synergistic reactions with other fibers. The use of a fiber-food supplement enables you to obtain adequate fiber from a wide variety of sources rather than excessive amounts from a single source. It's easy to get a heterogeneous selection of fiber in supplemental form. High-quality fiber supplements contain multi-fiber sources.

(5) Taking a fiber supplement on a regular basis assures an on-going weight-loss advantage on two counts:

a) *Because of the feel-full outcome.* As stated, chewing offers only a partial explanation for the satiating consequence of fiber. The other mechanisms involved are unknown, but several are possible.[14] Again: The water-holding properties of fiber make it likely that your gut contents are bulkier; distension of your stomach and small intestine helps induce satiety.[15]

b) *Because of fiber's lack of calories.* With supplementation, you can manage a high-fiber intake without adding significant calories—a double whammy to those extra pounds. It can't be overstated: Fiber is the only component in your daily diet that contains no calories, no fat, no cholesterol!

(6) Food sensitivities are dose- and frequency-related. Consuming small quantities of food substances, even those you are sensitive to, prevents food reactions from surfacing. So a scoop-full of fiber-food containing a variety of fiber is protective, especially when spaced several hours apart.

(7) Suppose you decide to have corn flakes for breakfast, a very low-fiber food. The glycemic index and insulin release will be greater than if you had a bowl of high-fiber cereal. If, however, you consume corn flakes with your extradietary fiber-food, the differences in these factors are hardly noticeable.[16]

(8) The unique benefits of rice fiber were described in Chapter 2. Average intake of fiber from rice is only moderate compared to other cereal-based diets. Yet we want the advantages of its health-giving active ingredients. Use of isolated rice fiber is an excellent idea. The same is true of several other fiber sources.

(9) Bran is only partially effective in restoring normal stool weight and transit time in patients who are constipated.[17] Again—taking a variety of fibers is much more effective.

(10) Because humans do not ingest foods singly, but rather as groups, a potpourri of fiber-food makes sense. In nutritional science, there is an increasing appreciation for the complexity of interactions of nutrients both in absorption and in metabolism, interactions which are beneficial.

The view that a single carbohydrate staple reflects a region's diet is not accurate. Most people—even isolated groups—consume multiple carbohydrate foods.

(11) Current attention to our changing environment emphasizes the need for protectors against the long-term influence of low-level radiation and means of removal of toxins from our bodies.[18]

> Nontoxic antioxidants (toxin destroyers), immunomodulators (substances which normalize the immune system), and adaptogens are part of the answer to environmental pollution. These are inherent qualities of fiber-food supplements.

(12) Fiber-food allows you to consume your fiber source with ease three or more times a day. Dependence on food alone for fiber sets you up for missing out on fiber intake when you eat at restaurants, get invited to dinner with friends, or open your fridge and find that no one has done the food shopping.

(13) Fiber supplementation and modification of fat intake are strongly effective in lowering cholesterol and triglycerides.[19] Taking a fiber-food supplement helps you to reduce your fat consumption, which in turn enhances the benefits of the fiber, which in turn expedites the reduction of cholesterol and triglycerides.

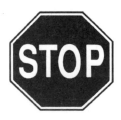

WARNING: Don't use your fiber supplement in lieu of good eating habits. Although a fiber supplement can be helpful, there is no substitute for natural, *intact* food.

THE FORMULA

A fiber-food supplement provides a way of getting a variety of fiber components in a utilizable, convenient form. As stated, such a supplement is usually derived from naturally-occurring plants and is offered as a mix of both soluble and insoluble fibers—a perfect symmetry of each variety of fiber necessary for optimal health. Manufacturers of quality fiber-food consider acid balance, swelling and gelling potentials, and water-binding capacities. The blend must be palatable, but not sweet (we don't want to undermine the benefits).

Formula Adjuncts

Calcium. A few well-designed fiber products contain calcium. Calcium is synergistic with fiber in protecting against colon cancer. The concern that fiber binds calcium has been raised. In general, however, the primary component of fiber, phytic acid, responsible for calcium binding has been found to be digested by bacteria in the colon. From there, the mineral can be absorbed. The ability for this process to occur is thought to increase progressively as your body accommodates to the addition of fiber.[20] Studies on mineral balance and high fiber diets demonstrate that mineral loss is not a problem. In fact, your body adapts to phytates very quickly, and phytates have been shown to reduce cancer risk.

Niacin-bound chromium. Recall that insulin increases the availability of glucose and decreases that of fat. Without chromium, however, insulin's powerful health-promoting properties (including fat-fighting) may be futile. Sadly, chromium is in short supply in the American diet. Excessive chromium losses are caused by food processing, inadequate dietary supply, refined sugar and other simple carbohydrates in the diet, exercise, and/or your body's inability to convert chromium to its biologically-active GTF form.

Supplementing with niacin-bound GTF-chromium contributes to weight loss because it potentiates insulin utilization, thereby reducing an overabundance of circulating levels of insulin. Because GTF-chromium can be a dietary counterpart in the reduction and control of body weight, it is a good adjunct to a fiber-food formula.[21]

Herbs. Because fiber supplements are designed to be bowel-cleansing, herbs may be added. Cascara sagrada, for example, may be included for its very slight laxative effect, or acacia for its soothing effect on the digestive tract—to name but two.

Miscellaneous Nutrients. Nutrients are synergistic. Don't be surprised if the fiber-product label reveals the presence of B vitamins, vitamin C, vitamin E, beta-carotene, omega-3, and so on.

Fiber-Food Supplement Facts to Consider

➤The maximum advantage of increased fiber is not usually achieved until approximately three months after starting consumption. During the first few weeks on a high-fiber supplement (or even foods with high-fiber content), increased abdominal distension and flatulence is not uncommon. You minimize stomach rumblings by increasing fiber slowly. Ignore recommended quantities, and begin with minuscule portions, adding gradually to the amount suggested. INCREASE FIBER INTAKE GRADUALLY.

➤If you are concerned about *too much fiber*, note this: The average transit time of South African schoolchildren on a high fiber regime is only nine and a half hours. Adding a fiber supplement to their diets reduces time only slightly. So if your fiber is acting maximally in respect to transit time (an unlikely occurrence for the average American), the addition of a supplement will cause no problem.[22]

➤Fiber supplements in powder form can be used in place of flour for gravies, sauces and dressings; in any shake; added to hot cereals. You can, for example, convert a stew to a high-fiber meal by adding supplemental fiber.

➤Extradietary fiber-food is likely to be most effective against the background of whole foods. That's why you should strive to consume foods in as natural a state as possible, and also take your fiber supplement a half hour before eating.[23] This curbs your appetite and helps to control your weight. If you are among the smaller percentage of people striving for weight gain (yes, such people do exist!), fiber-food works best after or between meals.

➤The aim is to slow gastrointestinal emptying for fewer or lower blood-sugar swings and to speed total transit time. Therefore, the ingestion of gastrointestinal stimulants such as wines and liquor with meals is likely to minimize the effectiveness of any fiber supplement.[24] If you are indulging, however, all the more reason to increase your fiber supplementation.

➤If fiber-food accompanies one meal, it has a positive health effect on your next meal, even if the subsequent meal does not contain fiber.[25] Such effects may be progressive with each successive fiber meal. This accounts for the longer-term health effects of the fiber.

➤If the reduction of processed fat has the same health benefits as increasing fiber, the latter is much easier to implement *in the form of a fiber supplement.* (Just think how much better off you will be if you can cut the fat as well!)

➤Avoid sizable feedings of a single fiber. Although it takes excessively large doses of any lone fiber to cause problems,[26] complexes of fiber-food prevent difficulties or sensitivities by offering small amounts of many fibers (as compared with large quantities of psyllium seed husk, for example). It may also be more appropriate to eat such fiber sources in quantities approximating that of their potential human dietary consumption, rather than very high quantities that would not normally be attained in human diets.[27] (Manufacturers of quality fiber-food supplements sold in the health industry consider these facts.)

➤For every extra gram of cereal fiber consumed each day, the average stool weight increases from 3 to 9 grams.[28]

➤Fiber absorbs copious amounts of water, so it's important to increase fluid intake along with a high-fiber diet. Taking any fiber supplement without adequate fluid may cause the fiber to swell before it arrives in your intestines.

False Alarms

From time to time, studies report that the digestibility of some nutrients decrease with an increase in the fiber content of the diet, which is believed to prevent the absorption of minerals.[29] This effect, however, has never been clearly defined. It may be that we sometimes compensate for the inefficiency of digestion and absorption with an increased secretion of digestive juices.[30] The effects of fiber must be considered in the context of the total diet and in the interactions of dietary components.[31]

Population groups who eat diets with a high concentration of fiber do not show clinical signs of mineral deficits.[32]

Scientists at the Institute of Nutritional Physiology in Karlsruhe, Germany, studied trace mineral absorption and fiber. They concluded that the binding of copper, zinc, and calcium to soluble fiber is extremely weak under the conditions present in the intestines. Minerals bound to fiber in the duodenum (the first portion of your small intestine) will be released again as they enter the jejunum and ileum (the middle and lower portions of your small intestine), where they still can be effectively absorbed through the intestinal walls.[33]

The cholesterol-lowering effect of the fibers that form gels occurs without compromising mineral balance in those who consume Recommended Dietary Allowance (RDA) levels of these minerals: calcium, magnesium, manganese, iron, copper, and zinc.[34] Since RDAs are generally low, it appears that mineral depletion from fiber is no cause for concern. Dr. Anderson, the diabetologist referred to earlier, has been following people for years, and finds that his recommended high-fiber diets, comprised of 50 milligrams a day, do not negatively impact on vitamin or mineral balance.

The presence of phytate, a water-soluble mineral-binding substance found in cereal fiber, has been regarded as disadvantageous. The fact is that phytates in legumes prevent blood sugar from taking its upward swing. Phytates also serve as antioxidants. Attaching to iron, they lower the danger of cancer-causing microorganisms in the intestines by grabbing their much needed iron supply.[35] It is becoming more apparent every day that the value of isolated fiber comes from more than just the fact that it's fiber.

SUMMARY

The totality of evidence links a high level of dietary fiber to health. Fiber carries a remarkably persuasive aura of disease prevention. But for any of these salubrious results to occur, the quantity of fiber consumed must be significant. Sheldon Hendler, M.D, on the faculty of the School of Medicine, University of California in San Diego,[36] encourages his patients to increase their fiber intake from what he observes is a typical 10 to 12 grams daily to 50 or 60 grams. "When I tell my patients to quadruple their fiber intake," says Hendler. "They look at me as if I've lost my mind. 'What do you want me to do?' a patient asked. 'Eat a bale of lettuce every day?'" (As you have learned, even if the patient consumed three heads of lettuce, the total amount of fiber would not exceed 5 grams.)

Are you ready to begin your fiber campaign? "Sometime" isn't ever *now*. This day will never come again (unless you're Shirley MacLaine). If you start today, you won't let disease creep over you. Along with diet changes, take your supplemental fiber-food NOW— show that you're made of tough fiber, literally.

Widespread use of high-fiber diets and/or fiber-food supplements will ultimately improve metabolic control and decrease health care costs for thousands of individuals; maybe even hundreds of thousands. We can decrease the size of our hospitals, but we won't do it by eating bran muffins.

My adrenalin still races when I read about studies similar to the apple/apple-juice experiments—published not only in medical journals, but now in the popular press. I am sorry for all the misleading Madison Avenue hype, but at least the world is noticing.

APPENDIX A

SUMMARY OF RESEARCH FINDINGS ON DIETARY FIBERS

Functions of Fiber	Fibers to look for in Supplements
Lowers serum cholesterol Soluble fibers are the best for lowering blood cholesterol levels.	*acerola fiber* *apple pectin* *barley fiber*
Speeds transit time Some fibers prevent metabolic waste and undigested foods from sitting in the colon for days and creating toxic by-products.	*beet fiber* *carrot fiber* *chickpea fiber*
Acts as a bulking agent Other fibers are good bulking agents. They absorb water and toxins in the colon and promote easier elimination.	*fig fiber* *flax seed fiber* *guar gum* *gum arabic*
Reduces blood sugar swings Certain fibers are important for people who are sensitive to low- or high-blood-sugar levels.	*gums (other)* *locust bean gum* *oat bran* *pectin*
Increases intestinal flora growth Fibers help the growth of healthful flora in the intestines, which aids in preventing the buildup of disease-causing bacteria.	*prune powder* *psyllium husks* *rice bran*

APPENDIX B

PERCENTAGE OF SOLUBLE AND INSOLUBLE FIBER

IN FIBER SUPPLEMENTS

FIBER SOURCE	SOLUBLE %	INSOLUBLE%	TOTAL
apple fiber	1.7	56.0	57.7
barley bran	3.0	62.0	65.0
beet fiber	24.0	50.5	74.5
citrus pectin	85.8	0.7	86.5
guar gum	90.0	0.0	90.0
locust bean gum	71.4	11.1	82.5
oat bran	15.0	3.2	18.2
pea fiber	21.0	65.0	90.0
prune fiber	5.7	3.8	9.5
psyllium husk	47.9	9.7	57.6
rice bran	7.7	20.4	28.1
soy fiber	5.2	71.2	76.4

Most fiber sources contain both soluble and insoluble fibers.

APPENDIX C

DIETARY FIBER IN POPULAR FOODS

Note: Quantities of fiber vary from chart to chart. This occurs because of variations in methods used for measurement and in different serving sizes. Since we don't go around measuring our food anyway, use these amounts as a loose, comparative guide.

FOOD	PORTION	GRAMS DIETARY FIBER
apple	small	2.8
apple muffin	1	1.0
apricot	1 whole	0.8
artichokes	1 large	4.5
asparagus	½ cup	1.7
avocado	½ average	2.8
banana	1 medium	2
beans (kidney)	1 cup	11
beans (lima)	½ cup	4.4
beets	½ cup	2.5
bread (white)	2 slices	1.0
bread (pumpernickel)	1 slice	1.3
bread (seven-grain)	2 slices	6.5
broccoli	¾ cup	5
buckwheat (kasha)	1 cup	9.6
carrots (raw)	4 sticks	1.7
carrots (cooked)	½ cup	2.3
cheese (any)	1 portion	0
chestnuts, raw (shelled, w/peel)	1 cup	14.5

chow mein	¾ cup	2
chickpeas	½ cup	6
corn on cob	1 medium	5
cucumber	10 thin slices	0.7
dates	2	1.2
figs (fresh)	1	2
grapefruit	½	0.8
green beans	½ cup	2.1
lamb chop	1	0
lentils	1 cup	6.4
lettuce	1 cup	0.8
matzo (meal)	1 cup	.2
milk	1 glass	0
mushrooms	4 large	2
oatmeal	½ cup	7.7
peach	1 medium	2.3
peanut butter	1 tbsp.	1.1
pear	1 medium	6
peas	½ cup	9.1
pineapple	½ cup	0.8
popcorn	1 cup	1
potatoes	1 small	4.2
prunes	3	1.9
raisins	1 tbsp.	1
raspberries	½ cup	4.6
rice (brown)	½ cup	5.5
rice (instant)	1 serving	0.7
sauerkraut	½ cup	1.5
spinach	½ cup	7
watermelon	1 thick slice	2.8
yams	1 medium	6.8

REFERENCES: AUTHOR'S NOTES

[1] Haines PS et al. "Eating patterns and energy and nutrient intakes of US women. *"Journal of the American Dietetic Association*, 1992 Jun, 92(6):698-704, 707.

[2] De Schrijver R; Fremaut D; Verheyen A. "Cholesterol-lowering effects and utilization of protein, lipid, fiber and energy in rats fed unprocessed and baked oat bran." *Journal of Nutrition*, 1992 Jun, 122(6):1318-24.

[3] Lovejoy J; DiGirolamo M. "Habitual dietary intake and insulin sensitivity in lean and obese adults. *"American Journal of Clinical Nutrition*, 1992 Jun, 55(6):1174-9.

[4] Howe GR et al. "A collaborative case-control study of nutrient intake and pancreatic cancer within the search programme. *"International Journal of Cancer*, 1992 May 28, 51(3):365-72.

[5] Heitman DW; Hardman WE; Cameron IL. "Dietary supplementation with pectin and guar gum on 1,2-dimethylhydrazine-induced colon carcinogenesis in rats." *Carcinogenesis*, 1992 May, 13:815-8.

[6] Musante L et al. "Hostility: relationship to lifestyle behaviors and physical risk factors. *"Behavioral Medicine*, 1992 Spring, 18(1):21-6.

[7] Watkins DW etal. "Magnesium and calcium absorption in Fischer-344 rats influenced by changes in dietary fibre (wheat bran), fat and calcium. *"Magnesium Research*, 1992 Mar, 5(1):15-21.

[8] Siddhu A et al. "Nutrient interaction in relation to glycaemic and insulinaemic response. *"Indian Journal of Physiology and Pharmacology*, 1992 Jan, 36(1):21-8.

[9] Sjodin P et al. "Effect of dietary fiber on the disposition and excretion of a food carcinogen (2-14C-labeled MeIQx) in rats. *"Nutrition and Cancer*, 1992, 17(2):139-51.

[10] Ferguson LR et al. "Adsorption of a hydrophobic mutagen to dietary fiber from taro (Colocasia esculenta), an important food plant of the South Pacific. *"Nutrition and Cancer*, 1992, 17(1):85-95.

REFERENCES: CHAPTER 1

[1] AMA Council on Scientific Affairs. "Dietary fiber and health." *Connecticut Medicine*, 1989 Sep, 53(9):529-34.

[2] Burkitt D. *Eat Right To Stay Healthy and Enjoy Life More*. New York, Arco, 1979, pp 9-10.

[3] Heaton W. "Food intake regulation and fiber," in *Medical Aspects of Dietary Fiber*, GA Spiller and RM Kay (eds). New York, Plenum Medical Book Co, 1980, p 224.

[4] Kestin M et al. "Comparative effects of three cereal brans on plasma lipids, blood pressure, and glucose metabolism in mildly hypercholesterolemic men." *American Journal of Clinical Nutrition*, 1990 Oct, 52(4):661-6.

[5] Ballmer PE. "Sense and nonsense of diets." *Journal Swuisee de Medecine*, 1990 Mar 17, 120(11):379-82.

[6] Ide T et al. "Contrasting effects of water-soluble and water-in soluble dietary fibers on bile acid conjugation and taurine metabolism in the rat." *Lipids*, 1990 Jun, 25(6):335-40.

[7] Drasar BS; Hill MJ. *Human Intestinal Flora*, London, Academic Press, 1974.

[8] Cummings JH. "Fermentation in the human large intestine: evidence and implications for health." *Lancet*, 1983, 1:1206-9.

[9] *National Cancer Institute*, 1987, 79(1):83-91.

[10] Wyman JB et al. "Variability of colon function in healthy subjects." *Gut*, 1978, 19:146.

[11] Harvey RF; Pornare EW; Heaton KW. "Effects of increased dietary fiber on intestinal transit time." *Lancet*, 1973, 1:1278.

[12] Walker ARP. "Effect of high crude fiber intake on transit time and the absorption of nutrients in South African schoolchildren." *American Journal of Clinical Nutrition*, 1975, 28:1161.

[13] Burkitt DP; Walker ARP; Painter NS. "Dietary fiber and disease." *Journal of the American Medical Association*, 1968, 229:1068.

[14] Eastwood MA; Mitchell WD. "Physical properties of fiber: A biological evaluation." In: *Fiber in Human Nutrition*, GA Spiller and RJ Amen (eds). New York, Plenum Press, 1976, p 109.

[15] Kamen B; Kamen S. *Kids Are What They Eat: What Every Parent Needs to Know About Nutrition*. 1983, New York, Arco Publishing, Inc, p 81.

[16] Longstaff M; McNab JM. "Digestion of fibre polysaccharides of pea (Pisum sativum) hulls, carrot and cabbage by adult cockerels." *British Journal of Nutrition*, 1989 Nov, 62(3):563-77.

[17] Agarwal V; Chauhan BM. "Effect of feeding some plant foods as source of dietary fibre on biological utilization of diet in rats." *Plant Foods for Human Nutrition*, 1989 Jun, 39(2):161-7.

[18] Hoppert CA; Clark AJ. "Digestibility and effect on laxation of crude fiber and cellulose in certain common foods." *Journal of the American Dietetic Association*, 1945, 21:157-60.

[19] Kay RM; Truswell AS. "Effect of citrus pectin on blood lipids and fecal steroid excretion in man." *American Journal of Clinical Nutrition*, 1977, 30:171.

[20] Tomlin J; Read NW. "Comparison of the effects on colonic function caused by feeding rice bran and wheat bran." *European Journal of Clinical Nutrition*, 1988 Oct, 42(10):857-61.

[21] McBurney MI; Thompson LU. "Fermentative characteristics of cereal brans and vegetable fibers." *Nutrition and Cancer*, 1990, 13(4):271-80.

[22] van Soets PJ; Robertson JB. "What is fiber and fiber in food?" *Nutrition Reviews*, 1977, 35:12.

[23] Costa MA; Mehta T; Males JR. "Effects of dietary cellulose, psyllium husk and cholesterol level on fecal and colonic microbial metabolism in monkeys." *Journal of Nutrition*, 1989 Jul, 119(7):986-92.

[24] McPherson-Kay R. Fiber, "Stool bulk, and bile acid output: implications for colon cancer risk." *Preventive Medicine*, 1987 Jul, 16(4):540-4.

[25] Cummings JH et al. "Colonic response to dietary fiber from carrot, cabbage, apple, bran, and guar gum." *Lancet*, 1978, 1:5.

[26] Ullrich IH. "Evaluation of a high-fiber diet in hyperlipidemia: a review." *Journal of the American College of Nutrition*, 1987 Feb, 6(1):19-25.

[27] Katan MB. "Direct and indirect effects of dietary fibre on plasma lipoproteins in man." *Scandinavian Journal of Gastroenterology*, 1987, 129:218-22S.

[28] Southgate DAT et al. "A guide to calculating intakes of dietary fiber." *Journal of Human Nutrition*, 1976, 30:303.

[29] Fairweather-Tait SJ; Wright AJ. "The effects of sugar-beet fibre and wheat bran on iron and zinc absorption in rats." *British Journal of Nutrition*, 1990 Sep, 64(2):547-52.

[30] Morgan LM et al, "The effect of soluble- and insoluble-fibre supplementation on post-prandial glucose tolerance, insulin and gastric inhibitory polypeptide secretion in healthy subjects," *British Journal of Nutrition*, 1990 Jul, 64(1):103-10.

[31] *National Cancer Institute*, 1987, 79(1):83-91.

32 Kamen B; Kamen S. *The Kamen Plan for Total Nutrition During Pregnancy*. New York: Appleton-Century-Crofts, 1981, p 180.

[33] Heaton, op cit,p 234.

REFERENCES: CHAPTER 2

[1] Kay RM and Strasberg SM. "Origin, chemistry, physiological effects and clinical importance of dietary fiber." *Clinical Investigative Medicine*, 1978, 1:9.

[2] Hoover-Plow J; Savesky J; Dailey G. "The glycemic response to meals with six different fruits in insulin-dependent diabetics using a home blood-glucose monitoring system." *American Journal of Clinical Nutrition*, 1987 Jan, 45(1):92-7.

[3] Baig MM; Cerda JJ. "Pectin: Its interaction with serum lipoproteins." *American Journal of Clinical Nutrition*, 1981, 34:50-53.

[4] Bobek P et al. "Effect of dehydrated apple products on the serum and liver lipids in Syrian hamsters." *Nahrung*, 1990, 34(9):783-9.

[5] Poynard T et al. "Reduction of post-prandial insulin needs by pectin as assessed by the artificial pancreas in insulin-dependent diabetics." *Diabetes and Metabolism*, 1982, 8(3):187-9.

[6] Hagander B et al. "Dietary fibre enrichment, blood pressure, lipoprotein profile and gut hormones in NIDDM patients." *European Journal of Clinical Nutrition*, 1989 Jan, 43(1):35-44.

[7] Morgan LM et al. "The effect of soluble- and insoluble-fibre supplementation on post-prandial glucose tolerance, insulin and gastric inhibitory polypeptide secretion in healthy subjects." *British Journal of Nutrition*, 1990 Jul, 64(1):103-10.

[8] Fairweather-Tait SJ; Wright AJ. "The effects of sugar-beet fibre and wheat bran on iron and zinc absorption in rats." *British Journal of Nutrition*, 1990 Sep, 64(2):547-52.

[9] Personal interview. Dr. Lester Packer, Ph.D., Department of Molecular and Cell Biology, University of California, January 1991.

[10] Gould, MN et al. "A comparison of tocopherol and tocotrienol for the chemoprevention of chemical induced rat mammary tumors." *American Journal of Clinical Nutrition*, 1991 April, 53(4):1068S-70S.

[11] Qureshi AA et al. "Dietary tocotrienols reduce concentrations of plasma cholesterol, apolipoprotein B, thromboxane B_2, and platelet factor 4 in pigs with inherited hyperlipidemias." *American Journal of Clinical Nutrition*, 1991 April, 53(4):1042S-46S.

[12] Ngah WZW et al. "Effect of tocotrienols on hepatocarcinogenesis induced by 2-acetylaminofluorene in rats." *American Journal of Clinical Nutrition*, 1991 April, 53(4):1076S-82S.

[13] Zhang JX et al. "The influence of barley fibre on bile composition, gallstone formation, serum cholesterol and intestinal morphology in hamsters." *Apmis*, 1990 Jun, 98(6):568-74.

[14] McIntosh GH et al. "Barley and wheat foods: influence on plasma cholesterol concentrations in hypercholesterolemic men." *American Journal of Clinical Nutrition*, 1991 May, 53:1205-9.

[15] Robertson et al. "The effect of raw carrot on serum lipids and colon function." *American Journal of Clinical Nutrition*, 1979, 32:1889-92.

[16] Jenkins, DJA et al, "Dietary fibers, fiber analogues and glucose tolerance: importance of viscosity," *British Medical Journal*, 1978, 1:1392.

[17] Kay, RM and Truswell, AS. "Effect of citrus pectin on blood lipids and fecal steroid excretion in man." *American Journal of Clinical Nutrition*, 1977, 30:171.

[18] Jenkins, DJA et al, "The cholesterol lowering properties of guar and pectin." *Clinical Science of Molecular Medicine*, 1976, 51:8.

[19] Lalor BC et al. "Placebo-controlled trial of the effects of guar gum and metformin on fasting blood glucose and serum lipids in obese, type 2 diabetic patients." *Diabetic Medicine*, 1990 Mar-Apr, 7(3):242-5.

[20] Turner PR et al. "Metabolic studies on the hypolipidemic effect of guar gum." *Atherosclerosis*, 1990 Mar, 81(2):145-50.

[21] Opper FH; Isaacs KL; Warshauer DM. "Esophageal obstruction with a dietary fiber product designed for weight reduction." *Journal of Clinical Gastroenterology*, 1990 Dec, 12(6):667-9.

[22] Behall KM et al. "Mineral balance in adult men: effect of four refined fibers." *American Journal of Clinical Nutrition*, 1987 Aug, 46(2):307-14.

[23] Truswell AS; Kay RM. "Bran and blood-lipids." *Lancet*, 1976, 1:367.

[24] Swain JF et al. "Comparison of the effects of oat bran and low-fiber wheat on serum lipoprotein levels and blood pressure." *New England Journal of Medicine*, 1990 Jan 18, 322(3):147-52.

[25] el Zein M et al. "Influence of oat bran on sucrose-induced blood pressure elevations in SHR." *Life Sciences*, 1990, 47(13):1121-8.

[26] Shinnick FL; Ink SL; Marlett JA. "Dose response to a dietary oat bran fraction in cholesterol-fed rats." *Journal of Nutrition* 1990 Jun, 120(6):561-8.

[27] Ney DM; Lasekan JB; Shinnick FL. "Soluble oat fiber tends to normalize lipoprotein composition in cholesterol-fed rats." *Journal of Nutrition*, 1988 Dec, 118(12):1455-62.

[28] Shinnick FL et al. "Oat fiber: composition versus physiological function in rats." *Journal of Nutrition*, 1988 Feb, 118(2):144-51.

[29] Mathur KS; Kahun MA; Sharma RD. "Hypocholesterolemia effect of Bengal gram: a long-term study in man." *British Medical Journal*, 1968, 6:30-1.

[30] Estevez AM et al."Supplementation of wheat flour with chickpea (Cicer arietinum) flour. II. Chemical composition and biological quality of breads made with blends of the same."*Archivos Latinoamericanos de Nutricion*, 1987 Sep, 37(3):515-24.

[31] Figuerola FE; Estevez AM; Castillo E. "Supplementation of wheat flour with chickpea (Cicer arietinum) flour. I. Preparation of flours and their properties for bread making."*Archivos Latinoamericanos de Nutricion*, 1987 Jun, 37(2):378-87.

[32] Hamberg O; Rumessen JJ; Gudmand-Hoyer E. "Blood glucose response to pea fiber: comparisons with sugar beet fiber and wheat bran." *American Journal of Clinical Nutrition*, 1989 Aug, 50:324-8.

[33] Carper J. *The Food Pharmacy*. New York, Bantam Books, 1989, p 254.

[34] Neal GW; Balm TK. "Synergistic effects of psyllium in the dietary treatment of hypercholesterolemia." *Southern Medical Journal*, 1990 Oct, 83(10):1131-7.

[35] Glassman M et al. "Treatment of type IIa hyperlipidemia in childhood by a simplified American Heart Association diet and fiber supplementation." *American Journal of Diseases of Children*, 1990 Sep, 144(9):973-6.

[36] Watters K; Blaisdell P. "Reduction of glycemic and lipid levels in db/db diabetic mice by psyllium plant fiber." *Diabetes*, 1989 Dec, 38(12):1528-33.

[37] Jenkins DJA. "Effect of eating guar and glucose on subsequent glucose tolerance." *Clinical Science*, 1979, 57:26.

[38] Lozano R; Chalew SA; Kowarski AA. "Cornstarch ingestion after oral glucose loading: effect on glucose concentrations, hormone response, and symptoms in patients with postprandial hypoglycemic syndrome." *American Journal of Clinical Nutrition*, 1990 Oct, 52(4):667-70.

[39] Costa MA; Mehta T; Males JR. "Effects of dietary cellulose, psyllium husk and cholesterol level on fecal and colonic microbial metabolism in monkeys." *Journal of Nutrition*, 1989 Jul, 119(7):986-9

[40] Seetharamaiah GS; Chandrasekhara N. "Studies on hypocholesterolemic activity of rice bran oil." *Atherosclerosis*, 1989 Aug, 78(2-3):219-23.

[41] Kamen B. "Innovative Supplements: Gamma Oryzanol and Ferulic Acid." *Health Foods Business*, 1990 Mar.

[42] Tomlin J; Read NW. "Comparison of the effects on colonic function caused by feeding rice bran and wheat bran." *European Journal of Clinical Nutrition*, 1988 Oct, 42(10):857-61.

[43] Topping DL et al. "Modulation of the hypolipidemic effect of fish oils by dietary fiber in rats: studies with rice and wheat bran. *Journal of Nutrition*, 1990 Apr, 120(4):325-30."

[44] Noronha IL et al. "Rice bran in the treatment of idiopathic hypercalciuria in patients with urinary calculosis." *Revista Paulista de Medicina*, 1989 Jan-Feb, 107(1):19-24.

[45] Gastanaduy A; Cordano A; Graham GG. "Acceptability, tolerance, and nutritional value of a rice-based infant formula." *Journal of Pediatric Gastroenterology and Nutrition*, 1990 Aug, 11(2):240-6.

[46] Hayes KC et al. "Lactose protects against estrogen-induced pigment gallstones in hamsters fed nutritionally adequate purified diets." *Journal of Nutrition*, 1989 Nov, 119(11):1726-36.

[47] Lo GS; Cole TG. "Soy cotyledon fiber products reduce plasma lipids." *Atherosclerosis*, 1990 May, 82(1-2):59-67.

[48] Lo GS et al. "Soy fiber improves lipid and carbohydrate metabolism in primary hyperlipidemic subjects." *Atherosclerosis*, 1986, 62:239-48.

[49] Madar Z. "New sources of dietary fibre." *International Journal of Obesity*, 1987, 11 Suppl 1:57-65.

[50] Tsai AC et al. "Effects of soy polysaccharide on postprandial plasma glucose, insulin, glucagon, pancreatic polypeptide, somatostatin, and triglyceride in obese diabetic patients." *American Journal of Clinical Nutrition*, 1987 Mar, 45(3):596-601.

[51] Bingham SA. "Mechanisms and experimental and epidemiological evidence relating dietary fibre (non-starch polysaccharides) and starch to protection against large bowel cancer." *Proceedings of the Nutrition Society*, 1990 Jul, 49(2):153-71.

[52] Iwane S. "Endoscopic study on the effect of dietary fiber against 1,2-dimethylhydrazine-induced colonic carcinogenesis in rats." *Japanese Journal of Gastroenterology*, 1989 Dec, 86(12):2713-20.

[53] Liu ZQ; Chao CS; Wu HW. "Investigation of the effect of a diet with wheat bran on the metabolic balances of Zn, Cu, Ca and Mg in diabetics." *Chung-Hua Nei Ko Tsa Chih Chinese Journal of Internal Medicine*, 1989 Dec, 28(12):741-4, 769.

[54] Anderson J; Tieryen-Clark J. "Dietary fiber: hyperlipidemia, hypertension, and coronary heart disease." *American Journal of Gastroenterology*, 1986 Oct, 81(10):907-19.

[55] Watts JM et al. "The effect of added bran to the diet on the saturation of bile in people without gallstones." *American Journal of Surgery*, 1978, 135:321.

[56] Schwartz SE et al. "Sustained pectin ingestion: effect on gastric emptying and glucose tolerance in non-insulin-dependent diabetic patients." *American Journal of Clinical Nutrition*, 1988 Dec, 48(6):1413-7.

[57] Fernandez ML; Trejo A; McNamara DJ. "Pectin isolated from prickly pear (Opuntia sp.) modifies low density lipoprotein metabolism in cholesterol-fed guinea pigs." *Journal of Nutrition*, 1990 Nov, 120(11):1283-90.

[58] Kay RM; Truswell AS. "Effects of citrus pectin on blood lipids and fecal steroid excretion in man." *American Journal of Clinical Nutrition*, 1977, 30:171-75.

[59] Hishinuma K et al. "Effects of intraperitoneally administered dietary fibers on superoxide generation from peritoneal exudate macrophages in mice." *International Journal for Vitamin and Nutrition Research*, 1990, 60(3):288-93.

[60] Ershoff B. "Antitoxic effects of plant fiber." *American Journal of Clinical Nutrition*, 1974, 27:1395.

[61] Finkel Y et al. "The effects of a pectin-supplemented elemental diet in a boy with short gut syndrome." *Acta Paediatrica Scandinavica*, 1990 Oct, 79(10):983-6.

REFERENCES: CHAPTER 3

[1] Hallfrisch J et al. "Continuing diet trends in men: the Baltimore Longitudinal Study of Aging(1961-1987)." *Journal of Gerontology*, 1990 Nov, 45(6):M186-91.

[2] Davis DL. "Natural anticarcinogens, carcinogens, and changing patterns in cancer: some speculation." *Environmental Research*, 1989 Dec, 50(2):322-40.

[3] Walker AR; Walker BF. "Appendectomy in South African inter-ethnic school pupils." *American Journal of Gastroenterology*, 1987 Mar, 82(3):219-22.

[4] Burkitt D. *Eat Right to Stay Healthy and Enjoy Life More.* New York, Arco Publishing, 1979.

[5] Walker AR; Seg AL. "What causes appendicitis?" *Journal of Clinical Gastroenterology*, 1990 Apr, 12(2):127-9.

[6] Friedman GD; Fireman BH. "Appendectomy, appendicitis, and large bowel cancer." *Cancer Research*, 1990 Dec 1, 50(23):7549-51.

[7] Larner AJ. "The aetiology of appendicitis." *British Journal of Hospital Medicine*, 1988 Jun, 39:540.

[8] Hughes RE. "Hypothesis: a new look at dietary fiber." *Human Nutrition: Clinical Nutrition*, 1986, 40C:81-6.

[9] Adlercreutz H et al. "Effect of dietary components, including lignans and phytoestrogens, on enterohepatic circulation and liver metabolism of estrogens and on sex hormone binding globulin (SHBG)." *Journal of Steroid Biochemistry*, 1987, 27(4-6):1135-44.

[10] Kato T; Takahashi S; Kikugawa K. "Loss of heterocyclic amine mutagens by insoluble hemicellulose fiber and high-molecular-weight soluble polyphenolics of coffee." *Mutation Research*, 1991, Jan, 246(1):169-78.

[11] Adlercreutz H. "Western diet and Western diseases: some hormonal and biochemical mechanisms and associations." *Scandinavian Journal of Clinical and Laboratory Investigation.* Supplement, 1990, 201:3-23.

[12] Van 't Veer P et al. "Dietary fiber, beta-carotene and breast cancer: results from a case-control study." *International Journal of Cancer*, 1990 May 15, 45(5):825-8.

[13] Rose DP; Connolly JM. "Dietary prevention of breast cancer." *Medical Oncology and Tumor Pharmacotherapy*, 1990, 7(2-3):121-30.

[14] Rose DP. "Dietary fiber and breast cancer." *Nutrition and Cancer*, 1990, 13(1-2):1-8.

[15] Brisson J et al. "Diet, mammographic features of breast tissue, and breast cancer risk." *American Journal of Epidemiology*, 1989 Jul, 130(1):14-24.

[16] Scott WN et al. "Levels of androgen conjugates and oestrone sulphate in patients with breast cysts." *Journal of Steroid Biochemistry*, 1990 Mar, 35(3-4):399-402.

[17] Adlercreutz H et al. "Diet and urinary estrogen profile in premenopausal omnivorous and vegetarian women and in premenopausal women with breast cancer." *Journal of Steroid Biochemistry*, 1989, 34(1-6):527-30.

[18] Holm LE et al. "Dietary habits and prognostic factors in breast cancer." *Journal of the National Cancer Institute*, 1989 Aug 16, 81(16):1218-23.

[19] Pryor M et al. "Adolescent diet and breast cancer in Utah." *Cancer Research*, 1989 Apr 15, 49(8):2161.

[20] Adlercreutz H et al. "Diet and plasma androgens in postmenopausal vegetarian and omnivorous women and postmenopausal women with breast cancer." *American Journal of Clinical Nutrition*, 1989 Mar, 49(3):433-42.

[21] Rosen M; Nystrom L; Wall S. "Diet and cancer mortality in the counties of Sweden." *American Journal of Epidemiology*, 1988 Jan, 127(1):42-9.

[22] Rosenberg EW et al. "Response to Crohn's disease and psoriasis." *New England Journal of Medicine*, 1983, 308:101.

[23] Reed BD; Slattery ML; French TK. "The association between dietary intake and reported history of Candida vulvovaginitis." *Journal of Family Practice*, 1989 Nov, 29(5):509-15.

[24] Story JA. "Dietary fiber and lipid metabolism." In *Medical Aspects of Dietary Fiber*, GA Spiller and RM Kay (eds). New York, Plenum Medical, 1980, p 138.

[25] Lowik MR et al. "Nutrition and serum cholesterol levels among elderly men and women." (Dutch Nutrition Surveillance System). *Journal of Gerontology*, 1991 Jan, 46(1):M23-8.

[26] Van Horn L et al. "Effects on serum lipids of adding instant oats to usual American diets." *American Journal of Public Health*, 1991 Feb, 81(2):183-8.

[27] Bell LP et al. "Cholesterol-lowering effects of soluble-fiber cereals as part of a prudent diet for patients with mild to moderate hypercholesterolemia." *American Journal of Clinical Nutrition*, 1990 Dec, 52(6):1020-6.

[28] Levin EG et al. "Comparison of psyllium hydrophilic mucilloid and cellulose as adjuncts to a prudent diet in the treatment of mild to moderate hypercholesterolemia." *Archives of Internal Medicine*, 1990 Sep, 150(9):1822-7.

[29] Wright RS; Anderson JW; Bridges SR. "Propionate inhibits hepatocyte lipid synthesis." *Proceedings of the Society for Experimental Biology and Medicine*, 1990 Oct, 195(1):26-9.

[30] Turner PR et al. "Metabolic studies on the hypolipidaemic effect of guar gum." *Journal Atherosclerosis*, 1990 Mar, 81(2):145-50.

[31] Lipsky H; Gloger M; Frishman WH. "Dietary fiber for reducing blood cholesterol." *Journal of Clinical Pharmacology*, 1990 Aug, 30(8):699-703.

[32] Ikeda I; Tomari Y; Sugano M. "Interrelated effects of dietary fiber and fat on lymphatic cholesterol and triglyceride absorption in rats." *Journal of Nutrition*, 1989 Oct, 119(10):1383-7.

[33] Kinosian BP; Eisenberg JM. "Cutting into cholesterol. Cost-effective alternatives for treating hypercholesterolemia. "*Journal of the American Medical Association*, 1988 Apr 15, 259(15):2249-54.

[34] Ullrich IH. "Evaluation of a high-fiber diet in hyperlipidemia: a review." *Journal of the American College of Nutrition*, 1987 Feb, 6(1):19-25.

[35] Anderson JW. "Dietary fiber, lipids and atherosclerosis." *American Journal of Cardiology*, 1987 Oct 30, 60(12):17G-22G.

[36] Beher WT; Casazza KK. "Effects of psyllium hydrocolloid on bile acid metabolism in normal and hypophysectomized rats." *Proceedings of the Society of Experimental Biology and Medicine*, 1971, 136:253.

[37] Fisher HP et al. "Dietary pectin and blood cholesterol." *Journal of Nutrition*, 1965, 86:113.

[38] Gubbins GP et al. "Collagenous colitis: report of nine cases and review of the literature." *Southern Medical Journal*, 1991 Jan, 84(1):33-7.

[39] Leo S et al. "Ulcerative colitis in remission: it is possible to predict the risk of relapse?" *Digestion*, 1989, 44(4):217-21.

[40] Polednak AP. "Knowledge of colorectal cancer and use of screening tests among higher-risk persons." *Journal of Cancer Education*, 1990, 5(2):115-24.

[41] Ferguson EF Jr; McKibben BT. "Preventing colorectal cancer." *Southern Medical Journal*, 1990 Nov, 83(11):1295-9.

[42] Willett WC et al. "Relation of meat, fat, and fiber intake to the risk of colon cancer in a prospective study among women." *New England Journal of Medicine*, 1990 Dec 13, 323(24):1664-72.

[43] Block JB et al. "Fecapentaene excretion: aspects of excretion in newborn infants, children, and adult normal subjects and in adults maintained on total parenteral nutrition." *American Journal of Clinical Nutrition*, 1990 Apr, 51(4):698-704.

[44] Cheah PY; Bernstein H. "Colon cancer and dietary fiber: cellulose inhibits the DNA-damaging ability of bile acids." *Nutrition and Cancer*, 1990, 13(1-2):51-7.

[45] Englyst HN et al. *Nutrition and Cancer*, 1982, 4:50-60.

[46] McLennan R. "Dietary fiber, transit time, fecal bacteria, steroids and colon cancer in two Scandinavian populations." *Lancet*, 1977, 2:2007.

[47] Reddy BSA et al. "Metabolic epidemiology of large-bowel cancer. Fecal bulk and constituents of high-risk North American and low-risk Finnish population." *Cancer*, 1978, 42(6):2832.

[48] Ferguson, op cit.

[49] Bingham SA. "Mechanisms and experimental and epidemiological vidence relating dietary fiber (non-starch polysaccharides) and starch to protection against large bowel cancer." *Proceedings of the Nutrition Society*, 1990 Jul, 49(2):153-71.

[50] Gorbach SL; Goldin BR. "The intestinal microflora and the colon cancer connection." *Reviews of Infectious Diseases*, 1990 Jan-Feb, 12 Suppl 2:S252-61.

[51] Skraastad O. "Dietary factors and risk of colon cancer." *Tidsskrift for den Norske Laegeforening*, 1990 Jan 10, 110(1):32-4.

[52] DeCosse JJ; Miller HH; Lesser ML. "Effect of wheat fiber and vitamins C and E on rectal polyps in patients with familial adenomatous polyposis." *Journal of the National Cancer Institute*, 1989 Sep 6, 81(17):1290-7.

[53] Sinkeldam EJ et al. "Interactive effects of dietary wheat bran and lard on N-methyl-N'-nitro-N-nitrosoguanidine-induced colon carcinogenesis in rats." *Cancer Research*, 1990 Feb 15, 50(4):1092-6.

[54] Nelson RL et al. "The effect of iron on experimental colorectal carcinogenesis." *Anticancer Research*, 1989 Nov-Dec, 9(6):1477-82.

[55] West DW et al. "Dietary intake and colon cancer: sex- and anatomic site-specific associations." *American Journal of Epidemiology*, 1989 Nov, 130(5):883-94.

[56] Roberts-Andersen J; Mehta T; Wilson RB. "Reduction of DMH-induced colon tumors in rats fed psyllium husk or cellulose." *Nutrition and Cancer*, 1987, 10(3):129-36.

[57] Finocchiaro C et al. "Role of diet in the treatment of constipation. Review of the literature." Italian. *Minerva Dietologica E Gastroenterologica*, 1989 Jul-Sep, 35(3):165-70.

[58] Johanson JF; Sonnenberg A; Koch TR. "Clinical epidemiology of chronic constipation." *Journal of Clinical Gastroenterology*, 1989 Oct, 11(5):525-36.

[59] Yakabowich M. "Prescribe with care. The role of laxatives in the treatment of constipation." *Journal of Gerontological Nursing*, 1990 Jul, 16(7):4-11.

[60] Marshall JB. "Chronic constipation in adults. How far should evaluation and treatment go?" *Postgraduate Medicine*, 1990 Sep 1, 88(3):49-51, 54, 57-9, 63.

[61] Schmelzer M. "Effectiveness of wheat bran in preventing constipation of hospitalized orthopedic surgery patients." *Orthopaedic Nursing*, 1990 Nov-Dec, 9(6):55-9.

[62] Liebl BH et al. "Dietary fiber and long-term large bowel response in enterally nourished nonambulatory profoundly retarded youth." *Journal of Parenteral and Enteral Nutrition*, 1990 Jul-Aug, 14(4):371-5.

[63] Finocchiaro C et al. "Role of diet in the treatment of constipation. Review of the literature." Italian. *Minerva Dietologica E Gastroenterologica*, 1989 Jul-Sep, 35(3):165-70.

[64] Cucchiara S et al. "Treatment of chronic functional constipation in children by administration of vegetable fiber (Dicoman 5.". Italian. *Minerva Pediatrica*, 1989 Mar, 41(3):147-52.

[65] Klurfeld DM. "The role of dietary fiber in gastrointestinal disease." *Journal of the American Dietetic Association*, 1987 Sep, 87(9):1172-7.

[66] Andersson H et al. "Transit time in constipated geriatric patients during treatment with a bulk laxative and bran: a comparison." *Scandinavaiaon Journal of Gastroenterology*, 1979, 14:821-6.

[67] Mann GV. "Diet heart: End of an era." *New England Journal of Medicine*, 1977, 297:644.

[68] Kestin M et al. "Comparative effects of three cereal brans on plasma lipids, blood pressure, and glucose metabolism in mildly hypercholesterolemic men." *American Journal of Clinical Nutrition*, 1990 Oct, 52(4):661-6.

[69] Anderson, op cit.

[70] Lo GS et al. "Effect of soy fiber and soy protein on cholesterol metabolism and atherosclerosis in rabbits." *Atherosclerosis*, 1987 Mar, 64(1):47-54.

[71] Kusni LH et al. "Diet and 20-year mortality from coronary heart disease. The Ireland-Boston Diet-Heart Study." *New England Journal of Medicine*, 1986, 312:311-18.

[72] Arnseymius AC et al. "Diet, lipoproteins, and the prognosis of coronary atherosclerosis. The Leiden Intervention Trial." *New England Journal of Medicine*, 1985, 313:805-11.

[73] Kromhout D. "Dietary fiber and 10-year mortality for coronary heart disease, cancer and all causes." *Lancet*, 1982, 2:518-22.

[74] Mundorff SA et al. "Cariogenic potential of foods. I. Caries in the rat model." *Caries Research*, 1990, 24(5):344-55.

[75] Grenby TH. "Snack foods and dental caries. Investigations using laboratory animals." *British Dental Journal*, 1990 May 5, 168(9):353-61.

[76] Peters P; Peters KM. "Fiber in the diet—certainties and speculation]." German. *Leber, Magen, Darm*, 1988 Jun, 18(3):156-63.

[77] Anderson JW; Ward K. "High-carbohydrate, high-fiber diets for insulin-treated men with diabetes mellitus." *American Journal of Clinical Nutrition*, 1979, 32:2312-21.

[78] Tsuji S; Wada M. "Diabetes Mellitus in Asia." *Excerpta Medica*, 1971.

[79] Trowell HC. "Dietary-fiber hypothesis of the etiology of diabetes mellitus. *Diabetes*, 1975, 24:762.

[80] Anderson JW et al. "Dietary fiber and diabetes: a comprehensive review and practical application." *Journal of the American Dietetic Association*, 1987 Sep, 87(9):1189-97.

[81] Leeds AR et al. "Meal viscosity, gastric emptying and glucose absorption in the rat." *Proceedings of the Nutrition Society*, 1979, 32:346.

[82] Jenkins DJA et al. "Dietary fibers, fiber analogues, and glucose tolerance: importance of viscosity." *British Medical Journal*, 1978, 1:1392.

[83] Kamen B. *The Chromium Diet, Supplement & Exercise Strategy*. Novato, California, Nutrition Encounter, 1990.

[84] Kestin, op cit.

[85] Fukagawa NK et al. "High-carbohydrate, high-fiber diets increase peripheral insulin sensitivity in healthy young and old adults." *American Journal of Clinical Nutrition*, 1990 Sep, 52(3):524-8.

[86] Khan HS et al. "Role of dietary fiber on platelet adhesiveness." *Journal of the Association of Physicians of India*, 1990 Mar, 38(3):219-20.

[87] Uusitupa M et al. "Effects of a gel forming dietary fiber, guar gum, on the absorption of glibenclamide and metabolic control and serum lipids in patients with non-insulin-dependent (type 2) diabetes." *International Journal of Clinical Pharmacology, Therapy, and Toxicology*, 1990 Apr, 28(4):153-7.

[88] Fernandez Soto ML et al. "Diet and non-insulin-dependent diabetes mellitus: historic and current perspectives]." *Revista Clinica Espanola*, 1990 Feb, 186(3):131-3.

[89] Morgan LM et al. "The effect of soluble and insoluble-fibre supplementation on post-prandial glucose tolerance, insulin and gastric inhibitory polypeptide secretion in healthy subjects." *British Journal of Nutrition*, 1990, 64:103-10.

[90] Roy MS et al. "Nutritional factors in diabetics with and without retinopathy." *American Journal of Clinical Nutrition*, 1989 Oct, 50(4):728-30.

[91] Tietyen J. Dietary fiber in foods: options for diabetes education. *Diabetes Educator*, 1989 Nov-Dec, 15(6):523-9.

[92] Schwartz SE et al. "Sustained pectin ingestion: effect on gastric emptying and glucose tolerance in non-insulin-dependent diabetic patients." 1988 Dec, 48(6):1413-7.

[93] *Annals of Nutrition and Metabolism*, as reported in *Vitamins and Minerals for Health*. Emmaus, Pennsylvania. Rodale Press, 1988.

[94] Mahapatra SC; Bijlani RL; Nayar U. "Effect of cellulose and ispaghula husk on fasting blood glucose of developing rats." *Indian Journal of Physiology and Pharmacology*, 1988, Jul-Sep, 32(3):209-11.

[95] Tsai AC et al. "Effects of soy polysaccharide on postprandial plasma glucose, insulin, glucagon, pancreatic polypeptide, somatostatin, and triglyceride in obese diabetic patients." *American Journal of Clinical Nutrition*, 1987 Mar, 45(3):596-601.

[96] Blackburn NA et al. "Mechanism of Action of Guar Gum in Improving Glucose Tolerance in Man." *Clinical Science*, 1984, 66:329-36.

[97] Leeds AR et al. "Guar Gum and Glucose Absorption: Absence of Evidence for Malabsorption." *Proceedings of the Nutrition Society*, 1978, 37:89A.

[98] Smith AN and Eastwood MA. "The Measurement of Intestinal Transit Time." in *Medical Aspects of Dietary Fiber*, GA Spiller and RM Kay (eds). New York, Plenum Book Co, 1980, p 31.

[99] Philipson H. "Dietary fiber in the diabetic diet." *Acta Medica Scandinavica*, 1983, 671:91-3S.

[100] Kiehm TG et al. "Beneficial effects of a high carbohydrate, high fiber diet on hyperglycemic diabetic men." *American Journal of Clinical Nutrition*, 1976, 29:895.

[101] Jenkins DJA et al. "Treatment of diabetes with guar gum: Reduction of urinary glucose loss in diabetics." *Lancet*, 1977, 2:779.

[102] Watters DA; Smith AN. "Strength of the colon wall in diverticular disease." *British Journal of Surgery*, 1990 Mar, 77(3):257-9.

[103] Brodribb AJM. "Dietary fiber in diverticular disease of the colon." In *Medical Aspects of Dietary Fiber*, eds GA Spiller and RM Kay, New York, Plenum Medical, 1980, p 46.

[104] Smits BJ; Whitehead AM; Prescott P. "Lactulose in the treatment of symptomatic diverticular disease: a comparative study with high-fibre diet." *British Journal of Clinical Practice*, 1990 Aug, 44(8):314.

[105] Chappuis CW; Cohn I Jr. "Acute colonic diverticulitis." *Surgical Clinics of North America*, 1988 Apr, 68(2):301-13.

[106] Wilson JL. "Diverticular disease of the colon." *Primary Care; Clinics in Office Practice*, 1988 Mar, 15(1):111-24.

[107] Brodribb, op cit, p 48.

[108] Morson BC. "Pathology of diverticular disease of the colon." *Clinical Gastroenterology*, 1975, 4(1):37.

[109] Eusebio EB; Eisenberg MM. "Natural history of diverticular disease of the colon in young patients." *American Journal of Surgery*, 1973, 125:305.

[110] Latto CRW; Wilkinson RW; Gilmore OJA. "Diverticular disease and varicose veins." *Lancet*, 1973, 1:1089.

[111] Fagin ID. "Does uncomplicated diverticulosis cause symptoms?" *American Journal of Digestive Diseases*, 1955, 22:316.

[112] Burkitt DP and Painter NS. "Dietary fiber and disease." *Journal of the Medical Association*, 1974, 229:1068.

[113] Cohen BI et al. "The effect of alfalfa-corn diets on cholesterol metabolism and gallstones in prairie dogs." *Lipids*, 1990 Mar, 25(3):143-8.

[114] Zhang JX et al. "The influence of barley fibre on bile composition, gallstone formation, serum cholesterol and intestinal morphology in hamsters." *Apmis*, 1990 Jun, 98(6):568-74.

[115] Hayes KC et al. "Lactose protects against estrogen-induced pigment gallstones in hamsters fed nutritionally adequate purified diets." *Journal of Nutrition*, 1989 Nov, 119(11):1726-36.

[116] Walker AR et al. "Prevalence of gallstones in elderly black women in Soweto, Johannesburg, as assessed by ultrasound." *American Journal of Gastroenterology*, 1989 Nov, 84(11):1383-5.

[117] McDougall RM et al. "Effect of wheat bran on serum lipoproteins and biliary lipids." *Canadian Journal of Surgery*, 1978, 21:433.

[118] Bergman F; Vanderlinden W. "Effect of dietary fiber on gallstone formation in man." *Z Erna*, 1975, 14:218.

[119] Jensen SL et al. "Maintenance bran therapy for prevention of symptoms after rubber band ligation of third-degree haemorrhoids." *Acta Chirurgica Scandinavica*, 1988 May-Jun, 154(5-6):395-8.

[120] Johnson CD; Budd J; Ward AJ. "Laxatives after hemorrhoidectomy." *Diseases of the Colon and Rectum*, 1987 Oct, 30(10):780-1.

[121] Anderssson H et al. *Human Nutrition: Applied Nutrition*, 1985 Apr, 39A:101.

[122] Burkitt D. "Fiber as protective against gastrointestinal diseases." *American Journal of Gastroenterology*, 1984, 79:249-52.

[123] Burkitt DP et al. *Lancet*, 1985 Oct, 2:880.

[124] Burkitt DP; James PA. "Low-residue diets and hiatus hernia." *Lancet*, 1973, 2:128-30.

[125] United States Bureau of the Census, *Statistical Abstract of the United States*, 1985, 105th ed, Washington, DC, 1984.

[126] Little P et al. "A controlled trial of a low sodium, low fat, high fiber diet in treated hypertensive patients: the efficacy of multiple dietary intervention." *Postgraduate Medical Journal*, 1990 Aug, 66(778):616-21.

[127] Anderson JW; Tietyen-Clark J. "Dietary fiber: hyperlipidemia, hypertension, and coronary heart disease." *American Journal of Gastroenterology*, 1986, 81:907-19.

[128] Burr, ML et al. "Dietary fiber, blood pressure and plasma cholesterol." *Nutrition Research*, 1985, 5:465-72.

[129] Wright A; Bursty PG; Gibney MJ. "Dietary fiber and blood pressure." *British Medical Journal*, 1979, 2:1541-3.

[130] Wright op cit.

[131] Hishinuma K et al. "Effects of intraperitoneally administered dietary fibers on superoxide generation from peritoneal exudate macrophages in mice." *International Journal for Vitamin and Nutrition Research*, 1990, 60(3):288-93.

[132] Kang ES et al. "Hepatic steatosis during convalescence from influenza B infection in ferrets with postprandial hyperinsulinemia." *Journal of Laboratory and Clinical Medicine*, 1990 Sep, 116(3):335-44.

[133] Leitch GJ et al. "Dietary fiber and giardiasis: dietary fiber reduces rate of intestinal infection by Giardia lamblia in the gerbil." *American Journal of Tropical Medicine and Hygiene*, 1989 Nov, 41(5):512-20.

[134] Painter NS. "Diverticular disease of the colon: the effect of a high fiber diet," *Royal Society of Health Journal*, 1975, 95:194-98.

[135] Cook IJ et al. "Effect of dietary fiber on symptoms and rectosigmoid motility in patients with irritable bowel syndrome. A controlled, crossover study." *Gastroenterology*, 1990 Jan, 98(1):66-72.

[136] Shankardass K et al. "Bowel function of long-term tube-fed patients consuming formulae with and without dietary fiber." *Journal of Parenteral and Enteral Nutrition*, 1990 Sep-Oct, 14(5):508-12.

[137] Friedman G. "Nutritional therapy of irritable bowel syndrome." *Gastroenterology Clinics of North America*, 1989 Sep, 18(3):513-24.

[138] Misra SP et al. "Long-term treatment of irritable bowel syndrome: results of a randomized controlled trial." *Quarterly Journal of Medicine*, 1989 Oct, 73(270):931-9.

[139] Prior A; Whorwell PJ. "Double blind study of ispaghula in irritable bowel syndrome." *Gut*, 1987 Nov, 28(11):1510-3.

[140] Fielding J; Kehoe M. "Different dietary fiber formulations and the irritable bowel syndrome." *Irish Journal of Medical Science*, 1984, 153:178-80.

[141] Manning AP et al. "Wheat fiber and irritable bowel syndrome: a controlled trial." *Lancet*, 1977, 2:417.

[142] Carter BS; Carter HB; Isaacs JT. "Epidemiologic evidence regarding predisposing factors to prostate cancer." *Prostate*, 1990, 16(3):187-97.

[143] Mills PK et al. "Cohort study of diet, lifestyle, and prostate cancer in Adventist men." *Cancer*, 1989 Aug 1, 64(3):598-604. Schelp FP; Pongpaew P. "Protection against cancer through nutritionally-induced increase of endogenous proteinase inhibitors—a hypothesis." *International Journal of Epidemiology*, 1988 Jun, 17(2):287-92.

[144] Adlercreutz, *Steroid*, op cit.

[145] Howie BJ; Schultz TD. *American Journal of Clinical Nutrition*, 1985, 432:127-34.

[146] Glise H. "Epidemiology in peptic ulcer disease. Current status and future aspects." *Scandinavian Journal of Gastroenterology*. Supplement, 1990, 175:13-8.

[147] Katschinski BD et al. "Duodenal ulcer and refined carbohydrate intake: a case-control study assessing dietary fiber and refined sugar intake." *Gut*, 1990 Sep, 31(9):993-6.

[148] Gimeno Forner L et al. "Antiulcerogenic properties of bran rice oil in rats." Spanish. *Revista Espanola de las Enfermedades del Aparato Digestivo*, 1989 Mar, 75(3):225-30.

[149] Jayaraj AP et al. "The ulcerogenic and protective action of rice and rice fractions in experimental peptic ulceration." *Clinical Science*, 1987 Apr, 72(4):463-6.

[150] Harju E; Sajanti J. "The protective effect of nutrients against stress induced gastric ulcers in the rat." *Surgery, Gynecology and Obstetrics*, 1987 Dec, 165(6):530-4.

[151] Rydning A et al. "Prophylactic effect of dietary fiber in duodenal ulcer disease." *Lancet*, 1982, 2:736.

[152] Dickerson JW et al. *Journal of the Royal Society of Health*, 1985 Dec, 105:191.

[153] Rosenberg EW et al. "Acne diet reconsidered." *Archives of Dermatology*, 1981, 117:193-5.

[154] Kaufman WF. "The Diet and Acne." *Archives of Dermatology*, 1983, 119(4):276.

[155] Putzier E. "Dermatomycoses and an antifungal diet." German. *Wiener Medizinische Wochenschrift*, 1989 Aug 31, 139(15-16):379-80.

[156] Klurfeld DM. "The role of dietary fiber in gastrointestinal disease." *Journal of the American Dietetic Association*, 1987 Sep, 87(9):1172-7.

[157] Harju E; Larmi TKI. "Efficacy of Guar Gum in Preventing the Dumping Syndrome," *Journal of Parenteral & Enteral Nutrition* 7 (1983):470-2.

[158] Morgan LM et al. "The effect of soluble- and insoluble-fibre supplementation on post-prandial glucose tolerance, insulin and gastric inhibitory polypeptide secretion in healthy subjects." *British Journal of Nutrition*, 1990 Jul, 64(1):103-10.

[159] Snow RC; Schneider JL; Barbieri RL. "High dietary fiber and low saturated fat intake among oligomenorrheic undergraduates." *Fertility and Sterility*, 1990 Oct, 54(4):632-7.

[160] Pederson AB et al. "Menstrual differences due to vegetarian and nonvegetarian diets." *American Journal of Clinical Nutrition*, 1991 Apr, 53:879-85.

[161] Woods MN et al. "Low-fat, high-fiber diet and serum estrone sulfate in premenopausal women." *American Journal of Clinical Nutrition*, 1989 Jun, 49(6):1179-83.

[162] Howe GR; Jain M; Miller AB. "Dietary factors and risk of pancreatic cancer: results of a Canadian population-based case-control study. *International Journal of Cancer*, 1990 Apr 15, 45(4):604-8.

[163] Mazur A et al. "Effects of diets rich in fermentable carbohydrates on plasma lipoprotein levels and on lipoprotein catabolism in rats." *Journal of Nutrition*, 1990 Sep, 120(9):1037-45.

[164] Ullrich IH. "Evaluation of a high-fiber diet in hyperlipidemia: a review." *Journal of the American College of Nutrition*, 1987 Feb, 6(1):19-25.

REFERENCES: CHAPTER 4

[1] Harlan WR et al. "Secular trends in body mass in the United States, 1960-1980." *American Journal of Epidemiology*, 1988, 128:1065-74.

[2] Guyton A. *Textbook of Medical Physiology* 5th ed. Philadelphia, WB Saunders Company, 1976, p 973.

[3] Desnoo K. "Des trinkende kind im uterus." *Monat. Geburt*, 1937, 105:88-97.

[4] Clydesdale FM. "Carbohydrate sweeteners in nutrition: fact and fantasy." In *Carbohydrates and Health*, LF Hood and EK Wardrip (eds). Westport, Connecticut: AVI Publishing Co., Inc., pp 128-32.

[5] Virkkunen M; Narvanan S. "Plasma insulin, tryptophan and serotonin levels during the glucose tolerance test among habitually violent and impulsive offenders." *Neuropsychobiology*, 1987, 17:19.

[6] Roland P; Augusto V. "Facilitating effect of insulin on brain 5-hydroxytryptamine metabolism." *Neuroendocrinology*, 1987, 45:267-73.

[7] Ashley D et al. "Evidence for diminished brain 5-hydroxytryptamine biosynthesis in obese diabetic and non-diabetic humans." *American Journal of Clinical Nutrition*, 1985, 42:1240-5.

[8] Sclafani A; Springer D. "Dietary obesity in adult rats: Similarities to hypothalamic and human obesity syndromes." *Physiology of Behavior*, 1976, 17:461.

[9] Kern PA et al. "The effects of weight loss on the activity and expression of adipose-tissue lipoprotein lipase in very obese humans," *New England Journal of Medicine*, 1990, 322:1053-9.

[10] Haber GB et al. "Depletion and disruption of dietary fiber. Effects on satiety, plasma-glucose and serum-insulin." *Lancet*, 1977, 2:679.

[11] Cleave TL. "The neglect of natural principles in current medical practice." *Journal of Research of the Naval Medical Service*, 1956, 42:55.

[12] Winnie G et al, "Effects of high carbohydrate diets on lipid accumulation in the rat. *American Journal of Clinical Nutrition*, 1973, 26:20.

[13] Haber, *Lancet*, op cit.

[14] Grimes DS and Gordon C. "Satiety value of wholemeal and white bread. *Lancet*, 1978, 2:106.

[15] Jordan HA. "Physiological control of food intake in man." In: *Obesity in Perspective*, GA Bray, (ed), Dept of HEW Publication No. (NHI) 75-708, Washington, DC, US Government Printing Office, 1975, pp 35-47.

[16] Rodin J. "Effects of obesity and set point on taste responsiveness and ingestion in humans." *Journal of Comprehensive Physiology and Psychology*, 1975, 89:1003.

[17] van Itallie TB. "Dietary fiber and obesity." *American Journal of Clinical Nutrition*, 1978, 31:S43.

[18] Nieman DC; Onasch LM; Lee JW. "The effects of moderate exercise training on nutrient intake in mildly obese women." *Journal of the American Dietetic Association*, 1990 Nov, 90(11):1557-62.

[19] Miles CW; Kelsay JL; Wong, NP. "Effect of dietary fiber on the metabolizable energy of human diets." *Journal of Nutrition*, 1988 Sep, 118(9):1075-81.

[20] Haber, *Lancet*, op cit.

[21] Anand BK. "Neurological mechanisms regulating appetite. In: *Obesity Symposium*, WL Burland et al (eds). Edinburgh, Churchill Livingstone, 1974, pp 116-145.

[22] Davis JD; Collins BJ. "Distention of the small intestine, satiety, and the control of food intake. *American Journal of Clinical Nutrition*, 1978, 31:S255.

[23] Rigaud D et al. "Overweight treated with energy restriction and a dietary fibre supplement: a 6-month randomized, double-blind, placebo-controlled trial." *International Journal of Obesity*, 1990, 14(9):763.

[24] Astrup A; Vrist E; Quaade F. "Dietary fibre added to very low calorie diet reduces hunger and alleviates constipation." *International Journal of Obesity*, 1990, 14(2):105-12.

[25] Deshaies Y et al. "Attenuation of the meal-induced increase in plasma lipids and adipose tissue lipoprotein lipase by guar gum in rats." *Journal of Nutrition*, 1990 Jan, 120(1):64-70.

[26] Astrup A, *Obesity*, op cit.

[27] Quaade F; Vrist E; Astrup A. "Dietary fiber added to a very-low caloric diet reduces hunger and alleviates constipation." Language: Danish. *Ugeskrift for Laeger*, 1990 Jan 8, 152(2):95-8.

[28] Levine AS et al. "Effect of breakfast cereals on short-term food intake." *American Journal of Clinical Nutrition*, 1989 Dec, 50(6):1303-7.

[29] Torsdottir I et al. "Dietary guar gum effects on postprandial blood glucose, insulin and hydroxyproline in humans." *Journal of Nutrition*, 1989 Dec, 119(12):1925-31.

[30] Mazur A et al. "Plasma and red blood cell magnesium concentrations in Zucker rats: influence of a high fibre diet." *Magnesium Research*, 1989 Sep, 2(3):189-92.

[31] Mezitis NH; Pi-Sunyer FX. "Dietary management of geriatric diabetes." *Geriatrics*, 1989 Dec, 44(12):70-2, 75-8.

[32] Porikos K; Hagamen S. "Is fiber satiating? Effects of a high fiber preload on subsequent food intake of normal-weight and obese young men." *Appetite*, 1986, 7:153-62.

[33] Krotkiewski M. "Effect of Guar Gum on Bodyweight, Hunger Ratings and Metabolism in Obese Subjects," *British Journal of Nutrition* 52 (1984):97-105.

[34] Anderson JW. "Dietary fiber and diabetes," in *Dietary Fiber in Health and Disease*. GV Vahouny and D Kritchevsky (eds). New York, Plenum Press, 1982, pp 151-65.

[35] Heaton W. "Food intake regulation and fiber," in *Medical Aspects of Dietary Fiber*. GA Spiller and RM Kay (eds). New York: Plenum Medical Book Co, 1980, p 236.

[36] van Itallie TB. "Dietary fiber and obesity." *American Journal of Clinical Nutrition*, 1978, 31:S43.

REFERENCES: CHAPTER 5

[1] Patterson BH et al. "Fruit and vegetables in the American diet: data from the NHANES II survey." *American Journal of Public Health*, 1990 Dec, 80(12):1443-9.

[2] Schapira DV. "The value of current nutrition information." *Preventive Medicine*, 1990 Jan, 19(1):45.

[3] Hand R; Antrim LR; Crabtree DA. "Differences in the technical and applied nutrition knowledge of older adults." *Journal of Nutrition for the Elderly*, 1990, 9(4):23-34.

[4] Berenson M et al. "Subject-reported compliance in a chemoprevention trial for familial adenomatous polyposis." *Journal of Behavioral Medicine*, 1989 Jun, 12(3):233-47.

[5] Slavin JL. "Dietary fiber: classification, chemical analyses, and food sources." *Journal of the American Dietetic Association*, 1987 Sep, 87(9):1164-71.

[6] Raymond LR et al. "The interaction of dietary fibers and cholesterol upon the plasma lipids and lipoproteins, sterol balance, and bowel function in human subjects." *Journal of Clinical Investigation*, 1977, 60:1429-37.

[7] Tinker LF et al. "Consumption of prunes as a source of dietary fiber in men with mild hypercholesterolemia." *American Journal of Clinical Nutrition*, 1991 May, 53:1259-65.

[8] Trainanedes K et al. *American Journal of Clinical Nutrition*, 1986 Sep, 44:390.

[9] McPherson-Kay R. Fiber, "Stool bulk, and bile acid output: implications for colon cancer risk." *Preventive Medicine*, 1987 Jul, 16(4):540-4.

[10] van Soest PJ; Robertson JB. "Analytical problems of fiber." In *Carbohydrates and Health*, LF Hood, EK Wardrip, and GN Bollenback (eds), Westport, Connecticut, AVI Publishing, 1977, p 76.

[11] Collier G; O'Dea K. "Effect of physical form of carbohydrate on the postprandial glucose, insulin and gastric inhibitory polypeptide responses in type 2 diabetes." *American Journal of Clinical Nutrition*, 1982, 36:10-14.

[12] Schneeman BO; Gallaher DD. "Dietary Fiber," in *Present Knowledge in Nutrition*, 6th ed, ML Brown (ed). Washington, DC: International Life Sciences Institute Nutrition Foundation, 1990, p 83.

[13] Wyman JB et al. "The effect on intestinal transit and the feces of raw and cooked bran in different doses." *American Journal of Clinical Nutrition*, 1976, 29:1474.

[14] Heaton KW. "Fiber, satiety and insulin—a new approach to overnutrition and obesity." In: *Dietary Fiber. Current Developments of Importance to Health*. KW Heaton (ed), London, Newman, 1978, pp 141-9.

[15] Davis JD and Collins BJ. "Distention of the small intestine, satiety, and the control of food intake." *American Journal of Clinical Nutrition*, 1978, 31:S255.

[16] Behme MT; Dupre J. "All bran vs corn flakes: plasma glucose and insulin responses in young females." *American Journal of Clinical Nutrition*, 1989 Dec, 50(6):1240-3.

[17] Muller-Lissner SA. "Effect of wheat bran on weight of stool and gastrointestinal transit time: a meta analysis." *British Medical Journal of Clinical Research Education*, 1988 Feb 27, 296(6622):615-7.

[18] Baraboi VA. "Radiobiology and the lessons of Chernobyl." Language: Russian. *Radiobiologiia*, 1990 Jul-Aug, 30(4):435-40.

[19] Lewis B et al. "Toward an improved lipid-lowering diet: Additive effects of changes in nutrient intake." *Lancet*, 1981 Dec, I.

[20] Persson I et al. "Effect of prolonged bran administration on serum levels of cholesterol, ionized calcium and iron in the elderly." *Journal of the American Geriatric Society*, 1976, 24:334-5.

[21] Kamen B. *The Chromium Diet, Exercise and Supplement Strategy*. Novato, California, Nutrition Encounter, 1990, pp 83-102.

[22] Walker ARP. "Effect of high crude fiber intake on transit time and the absorption of nutrients in South African Negro schoolchildren." *American Journal of Clinical Nutrition*, 1975, 28:1161.

[23] Jenkins DJA et al. "Effect of eating guar and glucose on subsequent glucose tolerance." *Clinical Science*, 1979, 57:26.

[24] Jenkins DJA. "Dietary fiber and carbohydrate metabolism." In: *Medical Aspects of Dietary Fiber*, GA Spiller and RM Kay (eds), New York, Plenum Medical Book Co, 1980, p 188.

[25] Jenkins, *Science*, op cit.

[26] Paulini I; Mehta T; Hargis A. "Intestinal structural changes in African green monkeys after long term psyllium or cellulose feeding." *Journal of Nutrition*, 1987 Feb, 117(2):253-66.

[27] Struthers BJ. "Warning: feeding animals hydrophilic fiber sources in dry diets." *Journal of Nutrition*, 1986 Jan, 116(1):47-9.

[28] Brodribb AJM; Groves C. "The effect of bran particle size on stool weight." *Gut*, 1978, 19:60.

[29] Suzuki T; Shimizu M; Ishibashi T."Proper energy evaluation of commercial laboratory animal diets based on digestibility and metabolizable energy values." Language: Japanese. Jikken Dobutsu. *Experimental Animals*, 1990 Oct, 39(4):557-64.

[30] Ikegami S et al. "Effect of viscous indigestible polysaccharides on pancreatic-biliary secretion and digestive organs in rats." *Journal of Nutrition*, 1990 Apr, 120(4):353-60.

[31] Kritchevsky D. "Fiber and cancer." *Medical Oncology and Tumor Pharmacotherapy*, 1990, 7(2-3):137-41

[32] Carrazza FR. "Minerals in Latin American diets." Language: Portuguese. *Archivos Latinoamericanos de Nutricion*, 1988 Sep, 38(3):599-621.

[33] Schlemmer U. "Studies of the binding of copper, zinc, and calcium to pectin, alginate, carrageenan, and guar gum in HCO_3-CO_2 buffer." *Food Chemistry*, 1989, 32:223-34.

[34] Behall KM et al. "Mineral balance in adult men: effect of four refined fibers." *American Journal of Clinical Nutrition*, 1987 Aug, 46(2):307-14.

[35] Graf E et al. *Cancer*, 1985 Aug, 56:717.

[36] Hendler, SS. *The Oxygen Breakthrough*, 1989, New York: William Morrow & Co., p 168.

INDEX